The Complete Dirty Talk 101 Collection

Featuring 20 Dirty Talk & Relationship Guides Anyone Can Use

Book 1

DENISE BRIENNE

Copyright © 2014 Denise Brienne

All rights reserved.

ISBN: 1499793804
ISBN-13: 978-1499793802

DEDICATION

This book is dedicated to anyone wanting to have better sex and better relationships.

Contents

101 BEDROOM TRICKS	8
101 CONFIDENCE BOOSTERS?	16
101 DAYS TO A GREAT SEX LIFE	23
101 DIRTY TALK EXAMPLES	32
101 DIRTY TEXT MESSAGES	39
101 EXTREME DIRTY TALK EXAMPLES	45
101 LOVE MAKING TIPS	52
101 MORE HARDCORE DIRTY TALK PHRASES	60
101 ONLINE DATING TIPS	67
101 PHONE SEX TIPS	76
101 PICKUP LINES	85
101 PLACES TO HAVE SEX	93
101 PLACES TO MEET SINGLE	99
101 SIGNS OF A CHEATING PARTNER	105
101 THINGS TO NEVER DO IN BED	113
101 ULTRA KINKY SEX IDEAS	120
101 WAYS TO CAPTURE HIS HEART	127
101 WAYS TO COME OUT OF THE CLOSET	134
101 WAYS TO FLIRT	141
101 WAYS TO MASTURBATE	149
HOW TO GET MORE DIRTY TALK	155
ABOUT THE AUTHOR	156

101 Bedroom Tricks

1. Blindfolds increase all other senses and make for an interesting experience.

2. Handcuffs are great for that "bad boy" routine.

3. Wear your high heels the entire time you're having sex.

4. Try out a new position every time you hit the sack.

5. Whisper your naughty fantasy into his ear - while you're in public. The wait to get home will be delicious torture!

6. Wrap your lubed hands around his penis and slide them back and forth, as if you were trying to start a fire with his…ummm…log.

7. Opt for flavored lube and use it generously for a slippery sensation.

8. Instead of rubbing your hands over your lover's skin, just tap with your fingertips.

9. Use a cock ring for even more girth from your man.

10. Strong mints with a dose of peppermint make for a tingly sensation on delicate body parts.

11. Don't stroke his penis - squeeze him rhythmically instead.

12. Moan your approval while you are sucking his dick.

13. Go down on him with a small piece of ice in your mouth?

14. Is he the adventurous type? Run that piece of ice along the crack of his ass while you give him head.

15. Draw the alphabet over her clit with your tongue.

16. Put on hot sex music and fuck to the beat.

17. Want to slow things down? Barry White makes for great lovemaking music.

18. Take a sip of ice water before going down; alternate it with a sip of hot tea.

19. Long day at work? Tie him up with his own tie.

20. Shave your body completely bare and put on a show for your lover.

21. Paint each other's bodies with a thin paintbrush dipped in chocolate sauce.

22. Dry-hump each other until you orgasm - with your clothes still on!

23. Always make eye contact.

24. Make short videos of you doing naughty things together.

25. Give a naughty massage from head to toe with scented massage oils.

26. Use a feather to touch your lover's body

everywhere.

27. Slip a piece of ice inside her and then go "fishing" to get it out with your tongue.

28. Get into the shower and get it on in the water.

29. Put a mirror beside the bed and watch what your sex session looks like.

30. Surround yourself with him in every way by wearing his cologne to bed.

31. Loop a pearl necklace around his cock and stroke him with it.

32. When she's fresh out of the shower, lick up every drop of water from her skin.

33. Let your lover watch your masturbate.

34. On the other hand, you could always watch him masturbate and tell him how to do it.

35. Do a striptease in the middle of the bed while your lover watches from underneath you.

36. Drape a red scarf over the bedside lamp for a sultry glow.

37. Explore the sensual heat of a good erotic spanking.

38. Slide your fingers as deeply into her as they will go.

39. Squeeze his butt while he slams into you in the missionary position.

40. Stroke him while wearing lubed latex gloves. The sensation will be surprising and fun.

41. On that same subject, why not try being the naughty nurse?

42. Invite your best friend to watch.

43. Or invite your partner's best friend to watch!

44. Come to bed in leather lingerie.

45. Use earplugs for utterly silent play - it's more intense than you think!

46. Take pictures of each other in the nude.

47. Introduce a vibrator into your sex play.

48. Use your fingernails to stroke his body from head to toe.

49. Let him watch as you suck your own nipples.

50. Have your ass lubed up before he comes to bed, and invite him to put his dick there.

51. Ask your lover to come all over your body.

52. Record the sound of your lover's orgasm on your voice mail so you can enjoy it anytime you want.

53. If you have long hair, drag it over your lover's body for a sweet sensation.

54. Put a porn movie on the television while you get it on. Imitate what the actors do.

55. Do nothing but kiss for ten minutes straight.

56. Climb on, put his dick inside you, and dance in place. The gyrations will amaze him!

57. Pretend to be someone else for an evening.

58. Fulfill a fantasy or two with your erotic toys.

59. Ask him to draw his name in an intimate place on your body with a Sharpie marker. Marking territory is hot!

60. Put lotion all over her body.

61. Switch your old cotton sheets with new satin ones.

62. Put her dildo in the refrigerator for a while and then slide it into her warm body.

63. Learn how to deep throat.

64. Play the "virgin" or "schoolgirl" to his "headmaster" or "sultan."

65. Read an erotic story to him while he strokes himself.

66. Lick his shaft and then blow cool air over it to give him shivers.

67. Leave the lights on during sex.

68. Have a glass of wine before bed to help you both relax and drop the inhibitions.

69. Ask him to detail his favorite fantasy while you

masturbate to it.

70. Are you truly adventurous? Invite someone home to join in with you.

71. Vow to go one week without sexual intercourse - only touching and kissing. The fun is in the trying!

72. Reach down and spank his ass while he's thrusting inside you.

73. When he's about to come, back off and squeeze the base of his penis until the sensation passes. Then rev him back
up. A few times of trying that and he will come harder than ever!

74. Pretend to be a prostitute and give your "John" whatever he wants.

75. Touch your lover only with your breath. Nothing else. See how long it takes before the begging begins!

76. Bring desserts to bed and offer your body as the plate.

77. Keep your panties on while you fuck - just move them to the side.

78. Play "20 Naughty Questions" while lying in bed together. Ask things guaranteed to turn up the heat.

79. Using Redi-Whip is an old cliché - but it works. Try it!

80. For the open-minded man, a strap-on can be a hot sex toy.

81. Set the alarm for thirty minutes early in the morning and use the extra time for sex.

82. Try the dice roll. Roll a pair of dice, and whatever number comes up is the number of minutes you will spend doing
whatever sex move he wants. Set a timer! When time is up, it's your turn.

83. Take the time to find her G-Spot. Believe me, it's worth the effort!

84. Practice your Kegel exercises so you can squeeze him while he's inside you.

85. Talk dirty to him with raunchy words you have never used before.

86. Drink your favorite wine from your lover's belly button.

87. Let your partner watch you undress. It's a simple way to turn them on!

88. Bite your lover gently all over their body. It's a unique sensation that doesn't happen every day!

89. Suck your lover's earlobe. You will be amazed at what happens.

90. Invest in soy wax body-friendly candles and drip the warm wax all over her body.

91. Offer to shave your lover's body before you make love.

92. Pretend to be a complete stranger and tell your partner wild things you want to try.

93. Kiss and suck on your lover's clean, bare toes. The sensation is incredible for man or woman!

94. Call a phone sex hotline, put it on speaker, and get it on while an invisible person urges you both to orgasm.

95. Suck on her fingertips until she's squirming for more.

96. Wake your lover up by going down on them.

97. Hop in the shower and wash your partner's body from head to toe - spending a great deal of time around their
middle, if you catch the drift.

98. Switch things up by doing it against the wall.

99. See how quickly you can engage in a quickie. Time how long it takes.

100. Try to stay completely silent during sex, while your lover tries to make you scream. The challenge can lead to serious fun!

101. Stare into your lover's eyes as you orgasm.

101 Confidence Boosters?

1. Have a hot, sexy romp in bed - all day long

2. Get a manicure and pedicure

3. Go to a bar and flirt outrageously with the cute bartender

4. Strap on a pair of high heels while doing the laundry

5. Wear your sexiest lingerie under your business suit

6. Have a one-night stand

7. Walk around the house naked all day

8. Make a list of compliments others have bestowed upon you

9. Talk to a friend about what you can do to boost your confidence

10. Have a "nooner" with your busy lover

11. Write a naughty story about you and your lover

12. Invest in that gorgeous dress

13. Buy weights and work out to the sound of your favorite music

14. Crank up that music and dance around the house

15. Make a list of the reasons you are successful

16. Go somewhere you have never been before

17. Think about the last time your lover worshipped your body

18. Take a course in something that interests you

19. Buy yourself a huge bouquet of flowers

20. Get an instant spray-tan for a healthy glow

21. Volunteer for your favorite charity

22. Get a haircut - something sexy and sassy!

23. Fake it until you make it

24. Turn up the radio in the car and sing at the top of your lungs

25. Buy yourself a new sex toy and use it immediately!

26. Take a pottery class

27. Turn to visualization - what do you really want? See it in your mind!

28. Keep a gratitude journal of the things that made you happy today

29. Get acrylic nails in a vivid color

30. Decide on what your purpose is. What drives you?

31. Start a blog and talk about your personal experiences

32. Have phone sex with a stranger

33. Leave a steamy message on your lover's voicemail

34. Take sexy pictures of yourself with a digital camera

35. Take a stripping class

36. Buy a nice gift for someone at work - for no reason at all

37. Go to a private beach in that new swimsuit

38. Have a makeover at the makeup counter

39. Rent a limousine for the evening

40. Go through your old high school yearbook and remember your first crush

41. Better yet, look up old high school friends and give them a call

42. Read old love letters

43. Take a walk - and smile at every stranger who crosses your path

44. Buy a drink for that gorgeous guy at the restaurant

45. Surprise your lover at the door in nothing but a sexy negligee

46. Wear a slinky evening dress to the local play

47. Get a thirty-minute shower…or a two-hour bath

48. Leave a huge tip for your waitress

49. Drop a nice check for a charity - anonymously

50. Set small goals for yourself

51. Surprise your lover with a new sexual move

52. Hop onto the internet and flirt in sexy chat rooms

53. Plan a private vacation for you and your honey

54. Buy a new perfume that makes you feel sultry and sexy

55. Pick one bad habit and resolve to stop - right now

56. Step out of character - walk the mall and pretend you're a celebrity!

57. Buy a pair of high heels much taller than what you usually wear

58. Leave a sexy note on a stranger's car

59. Then wear them to bed with your partner!

60. Visit your bookstore, buy a book about something new, and read it cover to cover

61. Sign up for aerobics classes

62. Better yet, hire a personal trainer

63. Read an erotic book while in the bathtub

64. Talk to a fashion expert about which clothes look

best for your figure

65. Go through your local drive-through…and pay for the order of the person behind you

66. Wear a barely-there thong

67. Plan a long night out with the girls

68. Eat dinner by candlelight

69. Clean up the clutter. This can make you feel so much better!

70. Give your old mentor a call and thank them for helping you get where you are today

71. Do the dishes in your underwear

72. Send your lover a letter - complete with a lipstick kiss

73. Have flowers sent to yourself at work - with no card, of course. Make everyone guess!

74. Learn how to give a lap dance, and then do it!

75. Start an email relationship with someone completely different from you

76. Make a list of reasons why someone should love you

77. Learn techniques for focusing, and apply them at work

78. Photoshop your own image into pictures with

people you admire

79. Rearrange your living room…or your bedroom

80. Learn a foreign language

81. Rent a convertible and cruise through your old neighborhood

82. Walk tall and straight, with perfect posture

83. Resolve to eat healthy foods and avoid the junk

84. Go somewhere you have always wanted to go

85. Spend a weekend simply pleasing your partner

86. Take a couple's cruise…or a single's cruise, depending upon your situation

87. Turn into a Mrs. Robinson and date a much younger man

88. Plan a movie day, and go by yourself. No sharing the popcorn!

89. Visit a spa and get a deep-pore facial

90. Invest in expensive moisturizers and use them religiously

91. Print out inspirational quotes and put them around the house so you see them every day

92. Listen to positive, upbeat music

93. Feeling brave? Take a turn at the strip club and

dance on the pole!

94. Make a point of living in the present

95. Meditate in a quiet room, with only the sound of your breathing for company

96. Make a list of things you love about your partner, and congratulate yourself on choosing so wisely!

97. Let go of a grudge and forgive the person who wronged you

98. Put up a personals profile and watch the compliments roll in

99. Have your photograph made by a professional photographer

100. Don't forget pets - their adoration is second to none!

101. Believe you're sexy…and you will be

101 Days To A Great Sex Life

1. Evaluate your sex life - do you like it?

2. Make a list of what you can do to change it.

3. Consider your background and your partner's background - how do they mesh?

4. Ask your partner to write down his wishes for your sex life.

5. What are your most impressive fantasies? Write them down.

6. Talk to your partner about them.

7. Start a gratitude journal. Write in it every day and explain what you love about your partner at that moment in time. Keep this up throughout the process…it comes in handy later!

8. What are your lover's favorite positions? Ask!

9. Read the Kama Sutra for tips.

10. Open up the "Dirty Talk" website and leave it up on the screen so your lover can see it.

11. Join the Dirty Talk forum to get new ideas.

12. Put away those old sweats and wear dresses around the house.

13. Go shopping for a new sex book together.

14. Get a makeover with a sexy new hairdo.

15. Send a card to his workplace - to his attention, of course.

16. Invest in new sheets for your bed.

17. Bring a dish of ice cream to bed with you and share it with him. No spoons allowed!

18. Send him a flirty text message…or two…or three!

19. Feeling even more adventurous? Visit the sex toy shop online.

20. Send flowers from a "secret admirer." Put the card in your own handwriting but don't sign it!

21. Buy a pretty new nightgown to wear to bed.

22. When he tries to put clothes on while you're home alone, tell him you want to see him naked.

23. Undress him when he comes home from work.

24. Meet him at the door with his favorite drink in hand and enjoy a few moments together.

25. Build up to great sex with one week of no intimate contact.

26. Invite your lover to touch you - but only with your clothes on.

27. Kiss your partner for five whole minutes.

28. Give him a massage without asking for anything in

return.

29. Go see a romantic movie together and hold hands.

30. Talk about the day you met and how far you've come since then.

31. Read a sensual story to each other in bed.

32. Plan a getaway weekend and purchase special naughty lingerie for the occasion.

33. Hop in the shower together and wash each other.

34. Commit to having sex for at least one long, luscious hour.

35. Plan on a weekend trip to the place you first met.

36. Leave the itinerary on his desk with a lipstick kiss.

37. Spray your perfume on the floorboards of his car - he will smell it when he gets in.

38. Tuck a sexy note into his briefcase or pocket when he's not looking.

39. Introduce him to breathing exercises. While you are lying in bed together, try to match your breaths to his. It becomes an intensely intimate experience.

40. Breathe the same air - cuddle up right beside him and take a breath when he exhales. Breathe from each other.

41. Compliment something about your lover that you have never complimented before.

42. Before you come to bed, casually run your fingertips all over your body - and make sure he can see you do it.

43. Write a sexy story about him, and then read it aloud in bed.

44. Call him for a lunch meeting at your favorite downtown hotel.

45. Give him a quickie when he gets home from work.

46. Let him find you soaking in the tub - with your waterproof vibrator in hand.

47. Surprise your lover with a naughty movie for the two of you to enjoy.

48. Tell your partner what you love the most about them.

49. Massage his shoulders as he sits and watches television.

50. Talk about what you both want out of life. What are your long term goals?

51. Watch the sunset or the sunrise together - your choice!

52. Pick up a treat for him at the grocery store.

53. Send a naughty picture of you through his private email.

54. Sit down and write "what I love about you" lists

Then exchange them and read aloud!

55. Give him hints about your perfect date night.

56. Eat at a fondue restaurant and feed each other every bite.

57. Make a list of why you fell in love with your partner in the first place, and then read it to them.

58. Invest in a lovely silk scarf...and use it as a blindfold.

59. Take a day for you. Get a manicure, visit the spa, whatever it takes to make you feel sexy!

60. Dance with your lover to a slow song on the radio.

61. Jump in the shower with him when he least expects it.

62. Purchase a nice lotion and take turns putting it on each other.

63. Ask for a list of the most creative sexual ideas your lover can think of - and then plan to act on them.

64. Talk about the "story of your life" - all the way to the happy ending.

65. Dedicate a song to your lover on their favorite radio station.

66. Write "I love you" in lipstick on the mirror before your partner wakes up.

67. Talk about what makes you happy. Not in bed - just

in a general sense. Ask your lover what makes them happy, too.

68. Write a letter to someone important in his life - his mother, his high school coach, his father, his mentor - and tell them how happy you are that they raised such a wonderful person.

69. Call your love and leave a steamy voice mail they can listen to over and over.

70. Surprise your lover at the office wearing a trench coat and nothing else. Does it sound like a bad porn movie? Maybe…but it works.

71. Invest in a book on how to improve your relationship and start reading it tonight.

72. Go out to a nice, romantic candlelit dinner. Agree not to discuss anything but each other.

73. Study up on feng shui and decide how to rearrange your living space to invite more sensuality in.

74. Go taste the wines at your local winery - or choose a few bottles and taste them yourselves at home.

75. Turn on loud music and dance your heart out. Invite your lover to join in!

76. Wear high heels around the house today.

77. Ask your lover for details about his childhood. Favorite pet? Favorite game? Whatever comes to mind is good.

78. Make a list of all the things you love about yourself.

Not your lover - about YOU. Tuck away the list in a drawer so you can look at it often.

79. Find a new sexual trick on the internet and break it out on your lover tonight.

80. Ask him to tell you a dirty story while you are in bed together.

81. Whatever you do today, hold hands and kiss often.

82. Spend a day away from your partner. Take the time to reflect on your relationship and how things are going.

83. Wake your lover up with kisses. No sex, just sweet kisses that make them smile.

84. Take some time today to learn about something your partner is interested in. For example, does he like football? Do you understand any of it? Today is the day to learn! Tell him what you learned when the evening rolls around.

85. Go to a museum or look at fine art online. What touches your lover?

86. Get inspired to create art of your own - invest in a few paints, some brushes, and a canvas. Draw something together and talk about what you are doing.

87. Now break out the body paints! Chocolate syrup, raspberry creams, even the old stand-by - whipped cream! - will look good on the canvas of your skin. Play until things get too hot!

88. Talk about trust and what it means to each of you.

89. Take a long walk together and talk about the one big regret in your life. Especially if you haven't shared it with anyone before. Tell your partner you trust them enough to say it out loud.

90. Break out of serious mode with some fun - what's the craziest position you can think of? Try it out tonight! Whoever is most creative wins a prize of their choice.

91. Break out the camera and take pictures of the two of you. Sweet pictures? Sexy pictures? That's up to you!

92. Remember the gratitude journal you started in the beginning? Show your journal to your lover.

93. Talk about barriers to intimacy. What makes you feel distant from your partner? How can you work on it together?

94. Choose a "secret word" that each of you will recognize as being a sign that you're turned on…but a sign that nobody else will ever recognize.

95. Have a quiet evening at home with no distractions. Make a romantic dinner and spend time on the couch watching a movie.

96. Ask your partner what feeds their soul. What drives them? What inspires them?

97. Sit down and plan your next vacation together.

98. Have a picnic in your own backyard.

99. When you see your lover today, go directly to him and give him the longest, biggest hug you can muster.

100. Watch your partner sleep.

101. Remember that it takes two, and it's never too late - so share this list with your lover and start all over again with the very first one!

101 Dirty Talk Examples

1. I love the way you kiss me…especially when you kiss me there!

2. I want to get naked with you right now.

3. Say my name when you do that!

4. I love you so much. Can you feel it?

5. Do you like the way that feels?

6. I love feeling your strong arms when you're on top of me. I love your muscles!

7. Use your mouth on me.

8. I love the things you do with your tongue.

9. You're so damn gorgeous.

10. What's that thing you do with your hand? I adore that!

11. Want to see what I really want? Come closer…

12. Strip for me, honey. Slow. I want to savor every inch of you.

13. Do you like the way that looks?

14. I'm going to control you tonight.

15. Use me as your toy.

16. Tell me what you want.

17. I'll do anything for a sexy lover like you…anything at all.

18. You're the best lover I have ever had.

19. This is going to be the dirtiest night of your life.

20. Show me what you can do. I know you're man enough!

21. You can have me any way you want.

22. Look, honey – handcuffs! What can we do with these?

23. Don't stop, harder!

24. You're the sexiest thing I've ever seen.

25. It drives me crazy when you look at me that way.

26. You know what I want. Give it to me.

27. I want you so bad – can you feel how much?

28. Just lie back and let me make you come.

29. You like that, don't you? You like it when your woman does that to you?

30. Look how ready I am. Don't you want to put your dick in there?

31. I adore how naughty you are.

32. You taste so good.

33. Come over here and ride me hard.

34. No one has ever made me come as hard as you can.

35. You make me so damn horny, baby!

36. I want to feel those sweet lips all over me.

37. Fuck me, honey. Right now.

38. I'm going to lick you and suck you until you come.

39. Want to make me scream? I'll bet you can.

40. Get over here, big boy. Show me what you're packing.

41. I love it when you nibble on my nipples.

42. Do that some more.

43. Your wish is my command.

44. Should I tie you up and make you take it, or are you going to be good?

45. Don't you dare come until I say you can.

46. I love how big your cock gets when I talk to you like this.

47. Fuck me with your big, delicious dick.

48. How deep can you go? Let's find out.

49. Lick every inch of me.

50. Only question is…where do you want to come?

51. How do you want me? On my knees? On my back? You choose.

52. Make me scream with that big dick of yours.

53. I'm going to suck you like a lollipop.

54. You give it to me better than anyone else ever could.

55. Do you like the way I fuck you, baby? Tell me.

56. Give me that big, fat baby-maker. You know what I want!

57. I'm going to do things to you that you've only fantasized about.

58. Give me that come, honey.

59. I want it in my mouth.

60. I want it all over me. Cover me with it.

61. Call me names. I love it when you call me your whore.

62. You can fuck harder than that. Give me everything you've got!

63. Make me scream like the naughty little slut I am.

64. Do you like it when I make you taste me?

65. I love sucking your rock-hard cock.

66. Tell me what you're doing. I want to hear the words.

67. Touch yourself. Let me watch you.

68. Can you see what you're doing to me?

69. Want a sex slave for the night? I'm yours!

70. Let's see how many times I can make you come. Want to place bets?

71. Tell me your most secret fantasy.

72. Do you like knowing you're the only one who fucks me?

73. How dirty can you get? How nasty are you?

74. Oh, yeah, baby…that's how I like to see it.

75. Watch me touch myself. I love it when you watch.

76. I want you to come in my mouth.

77. Shoot it down my throat.

78. You want to feel me come? Touch me right there – right now!

79. Tell me when, baby. I'll come with you.

80. How do I taste?

81. For the next hour, you're my personal sex toy. Deal with it.

82. Pound me with that hard, fat dick!

83. Better be careful…if you don't do what I tell you, I might stop.

84. What do you want tonight? The French Maid? The Hooker? The Schoolgirl?

85. Pretend you're a porn star. Fuck me like one!

86. I bet you would like to do this in public. Admit it.

87. Think I can swallow your whole cock? Let's find out.

88. I'm going to make you come until it hurts.

89. Play with my pussy.

90. Oh, God…that thing with your tongue. Do that again!

91. I love the way it sounds when you fuck me so hard. Hear it?

92. Tell me what you see. Describe it to me.

93. You like it when I spread my legs and take you in?

94. Come on, badass – show me how big a boy you really are!

95. You can have any hole you want. Which one will it be?

96. Do you want more? Take it!

97. Maybe you should spank me – I've been very, very bad.

98. Show me how a real man fucks.

99. Can you come again? I want some more.

100. I love getting dirty and naughty with you.

101. Do me like daddy use to do me!

101 Dirty Text Messages

1. i wnt 2 x u

2. i cnt w8 2 nuzzle ur nips

3. when will u b home in bd w/ me?

4. get off work early n cum get me

5. i wnt 2 lick u

6. i wnt 2 taste ur dick

7. i wnt 2 milk ur dick n get ur cream

8. i wnt 2 suck u

9. i wnt 2 lick ur cum from my fingers

10. get home so I can fuck u

11. r u hot yet?

12. r u hard already?

13. r u hot n bothered, baby?

14. r u warin nefin?

15. is ur dick long n hard n thick?

16. can anybody tell how hard u r?

17. r u gna show off ur cock?

18. r u naked?

19. do u wnt me?

20. u can hv me

21. all u hv 2 do is cum home n spread my legs

22. open me up wide 4 ur dick

23. i gna slide down ur hard cock

24. my puss is dripping wet

25. u can slide rite in

26. i wnt 2 ride on ur rod

27. i wnt 2 make u wet w/ my juices

28. i am 2uching myself rite now

29. wish u cud watch me!

30. on the bd w/o clothes

31. sliding my fingers inside my cunt

32. teasing w/ my nips

33. on the verge of cumin hard

34. my puss is so fucking hot!

35. i gna cum hard

36. i gna suck it gd

37. i just came 4 u

38. ram it in2 me

39. i ur dessert

40. suck me n I'll cum lyk crazy

41. u wnt 2 c my tits?

42. wnt 2 rub my puss?

43. i gna climb on 2p

44. slide my puss over ur cock

45. i gna ride u until u hv 2 cum

46. then Igna s2p

47. i gna give u a bj

48. ur gna shoot 4 me

49. cum all over my face

50. cum all over my tits

51. cum all over my puss

52. watch me play w/ ur cream

53. u wnt it dnt u?

54. when I c u I will get out the 2ys

55. i can take a 2y in each hole

56. u can fuck me wherever u wnt

57. dnt let anyone c ur naughty thots!

58. r u gna shr this text w/ ur friend?

59. would u lyk an orgy?

60. i do ur friend if u ask me nicely

61. can u imagine every hole full of cock?

62. u call the shots and tell me wut 2 do

63. wut do u wnt?

64. i wnt u 2 do me

65. i wnt u 2 give me all the fucking u can

66. when ur done I wnt u 2 turn me over

67. slide it up my ass

68. u wnt that tight ass?

69. make me feel lyk a virgin all over again

70. make me take it

71. make me take all ur friends

72. make me scream ur name

73. pump in2 me til u cum hard

74. make me cum hard, 2!

75. do u wnt 2 shoot it all over my face?

76. watch ur sticky crm slide down?

77. make me take it lyk the whore I am

78. u lyk having a slut 4 a luvr?

79. do nefin u wnt

80. i can do things u never imagined

81. i can make u feel btter than ne1

82. u wnt 2 treat me lyk a whore?

83. u can pay me lyk a slut

84. i wear high heels n fishnets

85. i give u wutever u wnt

86. u dnt hv 2 know my name

87. we can pretend Iur prostitute

88. wnt me 2 fulfill ur fantasy, baby?

89. u can watch me make it w/ ur bf

90. i can make it w/ my bf

91. i can fuck anybody u wnt

92. i can let u watch me fuck them

93. cum home and get me

94. ram ur cock hard in2 my puss

95. make me taste u in my throat

96. cum wherever u wnt

97. cum ne where

98. ur puss is w8n here 4 u!

99. my legs r spread and ready

100. hurry b4e I cum…

101. Do me w ur cock

101 Extreme Dirty Talk Examples

1. I want you to choke on my cock.

2. I'm going to piss all over you.

3. Fuck me like the whore I hired last night.

4. I'm going to blow a load in your ass.

5. You need to eat my cum, don't you?

6. All those other men lubed you up with their cum, didn't they?

7. Horny sluts always get what's coming to them.

8. I'm going to rape your ass.

9. Ride me like a fucking pony until I shoot into you.

10. Ripe me apart with your dick!

11. You like being gangbanged, don't you, slut?

12. I'll fuck you until you bleed.

13. If this how your daddy fucked you?

14. You fucked your mother like this, didn't you?

15. There's a reason they call you a motherfucker, you horny bastard.

16. Let me watch you fuck her.

17. Suck my cock after I've fucked your ass.

18. Drink down every ounce of that cream, baby.

19. Fuck me like a porn star.

20. Think I can fit my fist into your pussy? Let's find out.

21. You like being stretched by cocks, don't you?

22. I'm going to bit your tits until they bleed.

23. I'm on my period – so go down on me. Now.

24. Shut up and take it, you son of a bitch.

25. Bend over and spread your cheeks for my strap-on cock.

26. Real men know how to suck cock, don't they?

27. I'm recording all of this whether you like it or not.

28. I'm going to come all over you and let your boyfriend lick it up.

29. You're so horny you would fuck a dog if that were all you had around, wouldn't you?

30. I want you to wear a diaper for me.

31. I want to hurt you with my dick.

32. Shut the fuck up and take it.

33. I'm going to shoot my jizz all over your face.

34. What if I piss in your mouth? Would you like that?

35. I want to squeeze your balls until you shoot for me.

36. Suck your cream out of my pussy.

37. I'm going to fuck you so hard you scream.

38. Get down there and rim my ass.

39. Will you suck the milk out of my tits?

40. Here comes another load of cum for your ass…

41. Swallow my cum until you gag on it.

42. I want to watch you fuck a stranger.

43. I think you should pick up a woman at the club and anal fuck her.

44. I don't even know your name, and I don't care.

45. Are you crying? Good. That turns me on.

46. I want you to keep that butt plug in there until you are stretched enough to take my cock.

47. I'm going to tie you up and blindfold you before I fuck you.

48. I'm going to gag your mouth so you can't scream.

49. Then I'm going to pound your pussy as hard as I can.

50. And then I'm going to slam my dick into your ass.

51. You'll clean it all up with your tongue after I get off, won't you?

52. Jerk it until it hurts.

53. Stop whining, or I'll use Icy Hot instead of lube.

54. I've always wanted to do your mother.

55. Hell, I've always wanted to do my mother.

56. Come on, big sister – let's play!

57. I want to watch you get your dick pierced.

58. Let me suck on your high heels.

59. Put a collar on my neck and pull on it while you fuck me.

60. You feel like sloppy seconds, baby. Who did you fuck?

61. Do you know what a sounding rod is? Baby, you're about to find out…

62. I've always had a rape fantasy. You game?

63. Want to see me fuck your best friend? Want me to make you watch?

64. You would like to see me on my knees in a room full of men, wouldn't you?

65. I'm going to fuck you so hard you won't be able t

walk for a week.

66. Just how kinky are you? Should I shit in your hands to find out?

67. Wonder how he would feel to come home and see my dick in his wife?

68. Bark like a dog while I fuck you from behind.

69. Can't you spank me harder than that? Grow a pair!

70. I'm going to suck on your balls until they hurt.

71. Finger me while you're wearing your wedding ring – think your wife would approve?

72. I should put peanut butter on your dick and let the dog lick it off.

73. I love to watch my cum run down your thighs.

74. How much cum can you stand in that cunt of yours? How many men do you want?

75. I want to see some man-on-man action.

76. I want you to do my brother while I watch you.

77. Let's put clothespins on your nipples and see what that does for you, baby.

78. I want to watch you snowball with him.

79. How far can we stretch your cunt? Want to find out?

80. I'm going to pour champagne in your twat and suck it out.

81. Show me how you fuck your other lovers.

82. I'm going to lube your ass with my cum before he fucks it.

83. Can you taste my girlfriend's pussy juice on my dick?

84. Be careful or I might bite your clit.

85. Be a good girl for daddy and put on your play clothes.

86. What if I choked you while I fucked you?

87. A kinky slut like you deserves a belt across the backside.

88. Think we could fit a baseball bat up that loose cunt of yours?

89. Slide his dick in your ass, and then I'll fuck your pussy.

90. Put on a show, baby – you're live on the internet right now.

91. Let my cum on your face. I want to watch it ooze down your skin.

92. Put in a butt plug after I cum in your ass, so it stays deep in there all day.

93. What if you got a tattoo while I fucked you?

94. If you say no I will have to force you.

95. That makes you wet, doesn't it, you slut?

96. I want to fuck your dick so raw you bleed.

97. I'm going to give you an enema with wine and watch you get drunk.

98. Why don't you call your brother for a threesome?

99. I'm going to brand your ass with my initials while I fuck you.

100. I wonder if you can take my cock and this dildo up the same hole?

101. You're such a whore – are you sure you don't give it up for money?

101 Love Making Tips

1. Turn off the phone and lock the door - in other words, no distractions!

2. A little soft music always gets the mood going.

3. Invest in soft, comfortable sheets. Don't forget soft towels, too!

4. Candles give a soft, inviting glow to the bedroom.

5. Try slipping into a satin robe and showing a bit of skin at a time instead of the full Monty.

6. Kiss your lover for five minutes. That's right - FIVE! Not just a peck or a quickie.

7. Heat things up by reading a sexy story to your partner.

8. Talk about your fantasies. What do you want most?

9. Talk about fantasies you would never try, too. It's fun to share what's on your mind!

10. Give your partner a long, gentle massage.

11. Invest in massage oil candles - they heat up the oil just enough.

12. Better yet, try edible massage oil, so you can kiss your lover's skin while you caress it.

13. Choose your perfume or cologne carefully. Choose what you know your lover likes.

14. Don't talk about everyday life when you're in the bedroom. The bills and the kids can wait!

15. Try putting a colored light bulb into the bedside lamp. Red casts a sensual glow.

16. Be prepared with a small basket of necessities by the bed - lube, vibe, condoms, etc.

17. Blindfold your lover and make him guess what you're going to do next.

18. Lay back, put your hands over your head, and invite your lover to ravish you.

19. Pop a strong mint into your mouth before you go down on your partner - the better to tingle!

20. Keep a glass of ice water by the bed for refreshment.

21. You could also use the ice as a toy.

22. Try bondage! Use soft scarves if you're shy, handcuffs if you're not.

23. Watch a naughty video together and imitate what you see on the screen.

24. Challenge each other to be completely silent during sex. Place bets on who will speak first!

25. Challenge each other with dirty talk. Can you be filthy enough to make your lover speechless?

26. Use a rose to trace patterns all over your lover's

body.

27. Experiment with pillows to find new and interesting positions.

28. Breathe deeply with your lover - try to match the pace of your breathing with his.

29. Wear high heels to bed. Don't take them off!

30. Put on masks while you're making love and pretend you are other people.

31. Put soft gloves on your hands while you make love. Your partner will love the new sensation.

32. Slick your bodies with baby oil before you go at it.

33. Get silly - ask your Magic 8 Ball sexual questions.

34. Set up a digital camera to take shots of your lovemaking.

35. Want to be even more adventurous? Set up the video camera.

36. Place a mirror right beside the bed so you can see the action from different angles.

37. Put on deep red lipstick right before you go down on him.

38. Try out some flavored lubes or lubes made specifically for oral sex.

39. Perform a striptease. Use the bed post as your "pole."

40. Ask your lover to put on a striptease for you and praise his every move!

41. Perform in another way - masturbate for your lover.

42. Break out the vibrator and tease your lover with it.

43. Hop in the shower and make love in there - be careful of the slippery soap!

44. Invade the refrigerator. Whipped cream isn't just for pies, you know.

45. Whisper into your lover's ear after lovemaking.

46. If you have long hair, kneel over him and brush the strands all over his body.

47. Do you use condoms? Opt for flavored ones and try to guess the color.

48. Edible body paints turn your bodies into creative canvases.

49. Write erotic stories for each other and read them aloud.

50. Come to bed wearing leather - the surprise will turn him on!

51. Take it out of the bedroom. To the kitchen table, perhaps?

52. Give that backyard picnic table a shot - at night, of course, so the neighbors don't see.

53. Ask your lover to lie down and then touch him everywhere - with only one fingertip.

54. Go a step farther - touch him with only your breath.

55. Learn how to give a deep muscle massage and rock his world with your skills.

56. Shave your genitals for your lover. If he's up for it, shave his, too.

57. Put a temporary tattoo in a place where only your partner will see it.

58. Write your name on your lover's body with permanent marker.

59. Play strip poker - it's an old cliché, but hey, it works!

60. Look around your house for items that double as sexual objects. (Toothbrushes! Lotion bottles!)

61. Make love in the bathtub. The swirling water is a huge turn-on.

62. Role-play with your lover. Choose your parts and play them to the hilt!

63. Give your lover a paddle and ask him to spank you with it.

64. Make a point of foreplay - but without intercourse. Do this until you can't take it anymore.

65. Describe how your lover's body looks. Go into

great detail.

66. Get tipsy. Everything feels different after sharing a few drinks.

67. Take control. Drop to your knees the moment he walks through the door and suck him off.

68. Play "hide and seek" with a tiny piece of chocolate…make him explore your body to find it!

69. Ask him to take naughty pictures of you. Pose for him in your best lingerie.

70. Shop for toys together. You can do it online for privacy.

71. Explore what a cock ring does to him. Try it out in all positions!

72. Become his dessert plate. Arrange bite-size fruits on your body and let him feast.

73. Take a class in belly dancing and surprise your lover with your sensual moves.

74. Draw a "bulls eye" on your body with a pen and ask your lover to "hit" it when he climaxes.

75. Write down all your desires. Work down the list and fulfill one every night.

76. Hold your lover down while you make love to them. The possessiveness is a turn-on!

77. Look into a sex swing or other device that will make the bedroom a jungle gym.

78. Dress up for your lover in your finest attire - only to take it off one slow inch at a time.

79. Wear flavored body lotion to bed.

80. Run a feather all over your lover's body.

81. Offer your lover something you haven't done before.

82. Nibble on your lover's body. Start out gentle, but use more pressure if he really likes it.

83. Read through the Kama Sutra together.

84. Let your lover dress you - open your lingerie drawer and let him choose what you wear.

85. Wrap yourself in nothing but a big red ribbon and present yourself at the door.

86. Surprise your lover at work wearing nothing but a trench coat.

87. Let your lover watch you play with a vibrator or dildo.

88. Go online together and join an adult forum. Let your alter egos get down and dirty with others!

89. "Pick up" your lover at a bar and invite him back to the hotel room for steamy sex.

90. Record your sexual adventure and download it onto his MP3 player for later listening.

91. Make love standing up.

92. Go outside in a thunderstorm and have sex in the rain.

93. Learn exactly where to touch your man to give him the mind-blowing orgasm he really wants.

94. Learn a few dirty words in a new language and surprise him with your knowledge.

95. Use kitchen utensils for new sensations - the tines of the fork, or the whir of the whisk.

96. When he least expects it, dance for him in your underwear.

97. Challenge each other to having sex all day long. How many times can you come?

98. Invest in a remote controlled vibrator…and give him the remote.

99. Listen to audio stories together and try to mimic what is happening in the story.

100. Call a phone sex hot line and go down on him while the operator teases him.

101. Feeling brave? Invite a friend over to watch the action!

101 More Hardcore Dirty Talk Phrases

1. You're my naughty little bitch-slut, aren't you?

2. Get down on your knees and show Daddy that pussy.

3. Squirt that girl come on my dick, baby.

4. Pull it out and slam it hard.

5. Slam it so hard it bleeds, motherfucker!

6. Wank your dick while I watch you.

7. Stick that dirty cock into my slutty hole.

8. Suck your come off my dick, bitch.

9. Pump my cunt until I scream.

10. Fuck that whore until she screams. Just like that.

11. Come in my ass and then let me clean it off for you.

12. You want to feel my cream in your cunt?

13. Slam your man meat into my ass. Now!

14. Your ass is so pretty after I spank it all red.

15. I want to whip you while you're tied to the bed.

16. Come in me and then eat it out of me.

17. Lick my button with your hot tongue until I explode.

18. Squeeze my nipples until they hurt.

19. Watch me fuck your best friend. His dick is SO big!

20. You like fucking other women?

21. Spread my legs wide like the slut I am.

22. Damn, boy, you need to ream my ass like a motherfucker!

23. I'm a whore-slut. Punish me for it.

24. Let me clean my juices off your dick, Master.

25. Tease my clit with your cock. That's it.

26. Plow me until I can't breathe.

27. Think you can get your whole fist into my cunt?

28. I like to fuck you while your wife is watching.

29. You've got more girl meat than Tiger, don't you, manwhore?

30. Push your dick all the way into my throat.

31. Come hard while I can't breathe around your dick.

32. I want to feel your dick throbbing in my ass.

33. Fuck my ass while your best friend fucks my pussy.

34. I want to suck him while I fuck you.

35. Bite me while I come. Mark me.

36. Bang my ass with your fingers while I jack you.

37. Spread my ass out real good so I can take that monster dick up there.

38. Tie me up and make me fuck your buddies.

39. Fuck my high heels. Do it, bitch.

40. Watch your come slide down my legs.

41. Come in my pussy and then use the cream as lube to fuck my ass.

42. Do you like being a dirty whore?

43. I'll bet every guy in town has taken a ride up your chute.

44. Spread your legs and show me how many men have been in there.

45. You're nothing but a whore who eats come, isn't that right?

46. I'm going to suck on your balls while you fuck her.

47. I'm going to ride you while I suck him. Watch me baby.

48. I want to see you suck another man's dick. How much of a man are you?

49. Let's do it up the ass with a double dildo.

50. Damn, baby…I can taste that other bitch on your dick.

51. Squeeze your nipples and make them red for me.

52. That's it, honey. Spank that pussy. Spank it hard!

53. Suck my balls while I wank, you horny cumslut.

54. I'm going to stick my tongue in that little hole in your dick until you come all over it.

55. Come on her tits and let me lick it up.

56. Did she do you like this, you fucking cheater?

57. Watch me lick your come off my naughty, slutty hands.

58. Open up wide, cumbucket, here it comes!

59. Damn, girl…you're almost as good as your sister.

60. Force me down on your dick until I can't breathe.

61. You are going to come so hard you pass out.

62. I like fucking whores. You're number three tonight. Do you like that?

63. Feel my fingers in you? I'm going to push all of them in tonight.

64. You like doing that? My husband never sucks my pussy, but you do it soooo good.

65. How far can we stretch that slutty cunt? Let's find out!

66. I'll bend over and you can take my virgin ass with that dildo.

67. Shoot that cum into my mouth. Watch me swallow it.

68. Make me suck her clit for you while you fuck her.

69. You know what I want? Your dick. In my ass. With no lube. Go.

70. You like to have a string of men who just cum in you, don't you?

71. You're covered with the come of a dozen men.

72. Do you like the way it feels to slide through another man's come?

73. You like that? You like it when I finger your ass while I suck you?

74. I'm going to give you head until you can't come anymore.

76. Shoot that come all over my clit. See it dripping off, baby?

77. Pull out so you can see your come slide out of my pussy and lube up my ass.

78. I like blindfolding you. You don't know if that's a man or a woman sucking you off, do you?

79. That's it, honey. Jack off for us. You know we like to watch you.

80. You better not come for that slut. There will be trouble if you do, you fucking whore.

81. Shoot it in my face, you dirty bastard.

82. Shut up and lick my clit, fucker. Lick it harder!

83. Make me gag on your big dick.

84. Mmm…I love it when your cock stretches my asshole so tight.

85. You like rape fantasies? I'm going to fuck you until you scream and then fuck you some more.

86. I'm going to tie you up first so you can't make me stop, you fucking slut. You like that?

87. Spread your legs. That's right. Now touch your clit while I take a picture.

88. Take it all or I will slap the shit out of you, you goddamn pussy boy.

89. Feel my come in your throat? Swallow it. All of it.

90. Reach into your pussy with two fingers and jack me while I fuck your ass.

91. You do me so much better than my wife ever could.

92. Get me wet enough to fuck my ass with pussy juice.

93. I'm going to come all over your big dick!

94. You want hardcore, bitch? Piss all over my dick while I'm in you. That's just for starters.

95. I want to fucking eat your come for breakfast.

96. I'm going to fuck her ass and then make you clean me off. Whores do that, right?

97. Fuck me hard enough to make me pregnant, you stable stud.

98. You're nothing but a cum machine. That's what you are.

99. Stand up and jack off so all my friends can watch your dick explode.

100. Fuck my throat. I want to be so hoarse I can't talk.

101. You're going to have three dicks, one in each hole. Which one goes first?

101 Online Dating Tips

1. The most important rule: Be honest about who you are.

2. Use a good, current photograph.

3. Choose a dating site with a good reputation.

4. Investigate your dating service to decide if they are the right one for you.

5. It's okay to use more than one service at the same time.

6. Take your time in building your profile. It's the snapshot of your personality!

7. Be clear about what you want. If you only want a hookup, say so. Want more? Say so!

8. Use your profile heading to filter out the dates - for instance, "Looking for Younger Man" is a good way to get rid of those who are older than you.

9. Tell people how to contact you. Prefer email? Instant messaging? Make that clear.

10. There are free sites, but paid sites tend to provide more security.

11. Watch out for married daters, even if your site says they will weed them out.

12. If you are a serious stickler for privacy, give you photo only upon request.

13. Use a candid photo instead of a posed one - you will get more interest.

14. Use the message board on the dating site until you are comfortable with email.

15. Take the time to brush up on your communication skills.

16. Do not lie about anything - it will come back to haunt you!

17. Set up an email account that is meant only for online dating.

18. Don't become overwhelmed by an avalanche of interest. Choose carefully who will get a slice of your time, and tell the others - gently! - that you are too busy to keep in contact.

19. Don't give out your home phone number. Buy a disposable cell instead.

20. If you call them, use the "private" function on your phone to block Caller ID.

21. If someone emails you instantly and asks for your email, it might be a spammer.

22. If someone wants to move very fast, be wary!

23. Talk with potential dates via email until you are comfortable with a phone call.

24. The first phone call should feel natural. If it feels forced, think twice.

25. Don't discuss your children or family members by name - someone who really wants to uncover your real identity could use the names of your family to do it.

26. Keep the conversations about previous relationships to a minimum.

27. If anyone asks you to wire money, cease contact immediately.

28. If someone simply disappears after talking for a while, let them go. They might have found someone else, and they obviously weren't right for you.

29. If you get an unusual email that appears to be from a girlfriend or spouse, run fast and far.

30. If someone tells you they are "separated" get a firm idea of what that really means.

31. Is the picture they posted grainy or hard to see? That might be intentional, so avoid them.

32. Irregular or erratic responses usually indicate someone who is married or has something to hide.

33. If your potential date refuses to give you their phone number but insists on having yours, that's a big red flag!

34. Beware of someone who calls you at the same time every time. They might have a small window to call because they have another life to attend to.

35. Does your date never answer the phone but calls you back when it's convenient for them? That's not the

kind of person you want to be involved with.

36. Listen to your gut feeling. First impressions really are accurate!

37. If you had a great conversation or you love the emails, tell them so. Compliments are great!

38. The person you talk with should be friendly - not morose or angry.

39. Talk to friends and other dating site members about their experiences to weed out the bad apples.

40. If someone makes you feel great over the phone, you're probably on the right track.

41. Make note of what your date says - if they like Chinese, for example, that gives you a great lead on a wonderful first date.

42. Listen to what they have to say. Don't dismiss the more serious discussions.

43. On the other hand, don't fall for sob stories - you're not their psychiatrist!

44. If you have enough information on the person, run a background check.

45. If the person gets upset that you ran a background check, cut off contact with them.

46. By the same token, be understanding if they run one on you. You have nothing to hide, right?

47. If someone wants to make plans during odd hours,

be wary. They might be married.

48. Consider whether you want a long distance relationship before you look for partners outside your local area.

49. If you do decide to go for a long distance partner, make sure you and your potential partner are on the same page.

50. When it's time to meet, consider meeting halfway.

51. Uncomfortable about that much travel? Take a friend with you.

52. Whether you meet a long distance date or a local one, be clear about your intentions.

53. Do you want to have a relationship or just a hook up? Make sure your partner understands.

54. When you make plans to meet, agree to a very public place.

55. If they look completely different from their picture, walk away! Dishonesty is not a good way to start a relationship of any kind.

56. Tell your friends where you are going and leave a detailed itinerary.

57. Drive yourself to the location.

58. Have some sort of protection, such as pepper spray, just in case.

59. Better yet, take a self-defense class. It's good to do

no matter your dating situation.

60. Have a "safe call" - someone who calls you at a certain time to make sure you're okay.

61. Stay in a very public place throughout your first date.

62. Choose a very fun place, something you will both enjoy.

63. Dress appropriately for your date.

64. Stay confident! Confidence makes you oh-so-sexy.

65. Look for tan lines where a wedding band would be - this is a big tip-off to a married date!

66. Does your date answer his cell phone and conduct business as usual while he's with you? If you don't have his full attention, decline a second date and tell him exactly why.

67. If he seems shifty and keeps looking around for people who might recognize him, it could be more than just nervousness. If he calms down soon, fine - but if he gets more agitated, he could be afraid of being caught by someone!

68. Let the man make the first move when it comes to the kiss.

69. If you hit it off, go ahead and plan another date.

70. If you really hit it off and you choose to spend more time with them in private, let a friend know where you are going to be and how to reach you.

71. Thinking about having sex? Use condoms in addition to birth control!

72. Be prepared to never hear from the person again if you have sex on the first date. Many use dating services just to get laid.

73. Plan on meeting a friend at a certain time. If you don't show up after your wild night, your friend should be instructed to call the police. Better safe than sorry!

74. If your date pressures you to have sex, that is reason enough to end the relationship before it starts.

75. Want to see them again? Tell them so, but don't put any pressure on the decision.

76. Don't get possessive! When it's time to make your relationship exclusive, the topic will come up.

77. If he spends time with others from the dating service, take that as a sign that you can do the same - and if he has a problem with it, get rid of him!

78. If you know it's not going to work out, let your date down gently.

79. Never, ever disappear from someone's online life without giving a reason.

80. If someone disappears from your life without a reason, chalk it up to someone who was definitely not right for you in the first place.

81. Be honest about your reasons for not wanting to continue the relationship.

82. If you want to keep a friendship with them, tell them so.

83. If they don't want further contact with you, be understanding - after all, they are probably hurt by the loss of your potential relationship.

84. If your date doesn't want to see you again, take the news with grace and courtesy.

85. Don't break up over email or phone - do it face-to-face.

86. Hurt as little feelings as possible by making the breakup entirely about you - don't call them out on their shortcomings.

87. If you've been dumped, take the time to lick your wounds and rebuild your pride.

88. Don't "stalk" your former online love and try to figure out what is happening in their life now - just let them go.

89. If someone starts to stalk you, ask them to stop. If they don't, consider legal action.

90. Can you maintain a friendship with a potential date? You might be surprised at how many strong friendships have developed out of dating sites. Keep your eyes open to the
potential.

91. When you do find the person you want to be with, delete your profile.

92. If he doesn't delete his as well, it's a big red flag - be wary!

93. Cut your ties to those who are still hopeful to have a date with you. If you want to keep a friendship with them, say so - but don't give them further hope.

94. If you go through a breakup, don't immediately go back online. Take the time to heal.

95. Don't use online dating to make anyone jealous. It's deception of the worst kind for those who are looking for a potential mate.

96. Never tell someone you want to see them - but only if "this other person" doesn't work out.

97. If anything at all about your dating experience with a particular person makes you uncomfortable, get out of that situation immediately.

98. Be serious about online dating. There are real people and real emotions behind those profiles!

99. If things work out well for you, don't hesitate to tell people how you met. Meeting online obviously worked for you!

100. Treat everyone with respect throughout the entire dating experience.

101. Remember the golden rule: Always treat others as you would want to be treated!

101 Phone Sex Tips

1. Start out by telling your lover how much you want to fuck them - right now.

2. Talk about your hottest fantasy.

3. Read aloud from an erotic novel.

4. Sip some wine to get in the mood before you call.

5. Make certain the house is quiet and there are no interruptions.

6. Lock the doors!

7. Remind your partner of a naughty time together to get the fire started.

8. Tell how what you are wearing - and be honest.

9. Describe to him how you are undressing, piece by piece.

10. Let him hear as you spray perfume on your wrists.

11. Describe how it smells. Describe the room. Describe everything!

12. See phone sex as "painting a picture" in the mind of your partner.

13. Ask your partner to use props - maybe handcuffs around one wrist to symbolize your domination, or a candle to bring more intimacy to the room.

14. Wear a blindfold to enhance the experience of not being able to see your partner.

15. Drop your voice to a sultry growl.

16. Talk about what entices you most about your partner.

17. Ask your lover naughty questions.

18. "Confess" something you did in your past that you want to try again.

19. Keep ice chips nearby to keep your mouth moist while you talk.

20. Want to give him the blowjob experience? Suck a lollipop while he listens.

21. If you're the guy receiving the blowjob experience, use lots of lube to simulate saliva.

22. Ask your lover to describe their favorite fantasy scenario.

23. Use the postal service to help - send your panties through the mail so they are available and ready the next time you
and your lover have phone sex.

24. Don't be afraid to put the phone near your "private parts" so your partner can hear what you are doing with your
fingers.

25. Let your partner tell you how to touch yourself.

26. Watch porn together! Rent the same movie and start it on the same scene or time stamp. You can watch it together
from two separate places.

27. Tell your partner how you want them to come.

28. Try new positions - who says you have to be lying down while you get it on over the phone?

29. Remember everything your partner tells you so you can use it later, when you're together physically.

30. When you're ready for phone sex, get comfortable. Sitting in the kitchen chair might work for talking, but not for
getting it on!

31. Speak in a clear yet sultry voice.

32. Don't be afraid to get loud! Your partner will love it.

33. Carry the fun from one conversation to another. Start out with foreplay during the day and finish up at night.

34. Too tired to use a vibrator? The sound of your electric toothbrush works just the same.

35. Your moans are encouragement for your partner to keep talking.

36. Ask your partner what they are wearing. Trust me it works!

37. Tongue tied? Write a story in first person and rea

it aloud.

38. Wear that sexy lingerie to make the whole experience more realistic and fulfilling.

39. Experiment with your words. How explicit can you get?

40. Weave a fantasy so hot you have to stop talking. That's hotter than the fantasy itself!

41. If there is a word you don't like to use, simply don't say it.

42. If you prefer your partner doesn't say it, tell them gently - but not while you're in the heat of the moment.

43. Want to simulate being in the bathtub? Run water in your sink and slosh it around.

44. Send your partner a vibrator through the mail and ask them to use it while you listen.

45. Spank yourself for your partner - if they are into spanking, the fact that you are doing it to yourself will really turn
them on.

46. Use phone sex to explore your kinkiest desires, the ones you can't fulfill on a physical level.

47. Curse like a sailor if you're into it. It's a clue that you want to get more hardcore.

48. If he has a schoolgirl fetish, tell him about the new plaid skirt you're wearing.

49. If she has a need to be dominated, tell her about the new whip you just bought.

50. If you don't like the flow of the conversation, take charge and tell you partner what they are going to do.

51. Let your lover hear your orgasm. Don't hide a single bit of it.

52. On the other hand, playing around but agreeing not to orgasm is a fun twist!

53. Always say your lover's name, so they know you are truly into it with them.

54. You can be anyone when you're having phone sex, so have fun with roleplaying.

55. One of the best role-play phone sex games is the naughty telemarketer…you know you want to buy what he's selling,
don't you?

56. Don't be afraid to use your toys to simulate anal sex. Your partner will love it!

57. By the same token, sucking on a vibrator will sound just like sucking on a dick.

58. Sometimes act as though someone else is in the room, watching - and let your partner direct the action over the
phone line.

59. If you're the very open-minded type, have sex with someone while your phone sex partner listens in.

60. Better yet, call a phone sex hotline and conference it. You can both get off with a pro!

61. If you are in the same house as your partner, go into the bathroom with the cell phone and lock the door - then call
 them and have phone sex. It's a fun twist on the same old sex routine!

62. Describe everything your body is doing - nipples hard, breathing hard, etc.

63. Try to reach orgasm at the same time.

64. Call your lover sexy names, like slut or whore.

65. Let your partner give you instructions before you have phone sex. You might be told to wear a cock ring while you
 wait for the call, or to use a dildo to get you wet before he rings you up.

66. Don't come until your partner gives you the "okay."

67. Smile when you talk - it makes your voice sound happier.

68. Give your lover dares, like masturbating with the windows open.

69. Send photographs of your sexiest lingerie to feed his phone sex fantasies.

70. Simply listen to your partner masturbate until orgasm - and then do the same for them. The act of listening and not
 talking at all can enhance the experience.

71. Tell them how turned on you are.

72. Ask them what they want you to do to yourself. Tell them it can be anything!

73. Use sex toys, like nipple clamps, to heighten sensation when talking about a BDSM fantasy.

74. Let your phone sex partner hear the sound of your vibrator sliding in and out of you.

75. Spice it up with naughty text messages during the day.

76. Want to make phone sex hotter? Use a webcam.

77. If you're on the kinky side, jack off on something - or in something - and send it to your lover.

78. Don't be afraid to taste yourself - your partner will love the sound of that.

79. Tell them how much you love their voice.

80. If they have a filthy mind, tell them so - and ask them to tell you more.

81. Tell your partner what you are going to do to them the next time you see them. Keep it real - you might be asked to
deliver!

82. Put on hot music in the background and tell your partner you want to fuck to the beat.

83. Send your male partner a "pocket pussy" to engage

in phone sex fantasies with you.

84. Don't forget to laugh - phone sex should be fun!

85. If you're having phone sex with a stranger, get your own orgasm first - it's sad to say, but many people will cut and
run after they get theirs, and you don't want that!

86. If you're open-minded, have phone sex in front of your friends.

87. Have phone sex with someone across a crowded bar - you can't see them, but you can hear them, and it's a huge
turn-on.

88. Videotape yourself having phone sex with your partner, then send it to them.

89. Make an audio recording of you getting off to your partner's words.

90. Don't want to cheat on your partner but need more spice in your life? Have phone sex with someone else.

91. Set a "date" for phone sex and make it stretch out for two or three hours.

92. Tease your partner with your orgasm when they are in a place where phone sex is not a good idea - like when they
are driving, or in a business meeting.

93. Tell your partner you have just shaved your private parts, and describe how slick they are now that you are aroused

for them.

94. Jump on a phone sex chat line for spur-of-the-moment ideas.

95. Does your phone have a good speaker? Have phone sex in the shower.

96. Go to a public place and get it on over the phone. Make it a place your partner knows, so you can have a memory to
share.

97. Kiss your hand near the phone for the perfect sound of kisses on your partner's skin.

98. Use the hottest dirty talk phrases you can imagine.

99. Spin a naughty fantasy that you could not possibly act out in real life.

100. Tell your partner exactly how you are touching yourself.

101. Remember to say "thank you" for letting you listen to their most intimate moments.

101 Pickup Lines

1. So, do you come here often?

2. What's your sign?

3. Did it hurt? Did it hurt when you fell from heaven?

4. You must be tired, because you've been running through my mind all day.

5. My mother has been praying I would bring home a girl like you.

6. May I buy you a drink?

7. I know a great way to burn off all these calories.

8. What will it take to make you sleep with me? I'm listening.

9. Can I take your coat…or would you like to help me put one on?

10. I want to wake up next to you in the morning.

11. Can I give you a ride home?

12. I'll bet you a hundred bucks you're going to say no.

13. Your place or mine?

14. No, I haven't been drinking. I'm just intoxicated by your beauty.

15. The stars fell from the sky and landed in your eyes.

16. My wife just left me for another man. Want to help me get even?

17. Let's go someplace quieter - I really want to hear what you have to say.

18. Your beauty makes the rest of the world look sad and gray.

19. Looking that sexy has got to be a crime in at least forty states.

20. I saw you looking at me. Do you want me?

21. You're so beautiful, I don't remember a single pickup line.

22. Besides being sexy all the time, what do you do for a living?

23. If I'm dreaming, please don't wake me up.

24. I want to file a police report. You just stole my heart.

25. I know you're from heaven - but where do you spend your time on Earth?

26. I was surprised the fire alarms didn't go off when your hotness walked in.

27. Are you from Tennessee? You're the only ten I see.

28. Excuse me while I pick my jaw up from the floor.

29. Don't turn your back on me - I might have to st

your heart.

30. I saw your picture in the dictionary next to the word "hot."

31. I've lost my phone number. Can I have yours?

32. Oh, my…there really are angels among us. How long are you here?

33. Are you afraid of commitment? No? Prove it.

34. Can I take your puppies out to play?

35. I must be dead. Beauties like you are only possible in heaven.

36. That's a gorgeous dress. Can I talk you out of it?

37. Do you want children? How about we practice making them?

38. Fuck me if I'm wrong, but is your name Stacy?

39. Did you ever win "best in show"? You're definitely a winner.

40. It's not fair that you get that body for the rest of your life. Can you share it for just one night?

41. I thought I needed Viagra…and then I saw you.

42. Those pants are so clean, I can see myself in them.

43. You're so bad, you broke Santa's naughty list!

44. Ever do it with a stranger? Tonight's your lucky

night!

45. I'm not good at breaking the ice, so I'll just say hello instead.

46. I really do melt in your mouth, not in your hand.

47. If not for all that sin, you would be perfect.

48. Who needs a horse race when a Thoroughbred like you is sitting right here?

49. Will you hold my hand while I go for a walk? Come on.

50. I'm Latino. Do you have any Latino in you? Want some?

51. I'll bet you don't have the energy to keep up with me. Let's go find out.

52. What does it feel like to be the sexiest person in the room?

53. I'm going to get off on you tonight anyway - you might as well be there while I do it.

54. We're going to dance, then drink, then fuck. You okay with that?

55. I think I'm falling in love with you.

56. I tried being a monk, but celibacy just isn't my style.

57. You know how to give CPR? My dick needs some air - how about mouth to mouth?

58. My backseat is the size of a football field. Want to see?

59. I have much more money than you think.

60. You have a headache? You know what cures that, don't you?

61. Those legs go on for miles and miles…can I drive them?

62. I just got out of prison and I haven't had a woman in years. Want to make up for it?

63. What do you like for breakfast?

64. Your lips look lonely…I can give them something to do.

65. Excuse me…I think you have my chair.

66. Are you married? You are? You didn't say happily, so I still have a chance.

67. I was a Boy Scout, honey - you should see what I can do with some rope.

68. I'm a gynecologist. How long has it been since your last exam?

69. Don't you think we would look gorgeous in an engagement photo?

70. When is the last time you were kissed?

71. Are you a virgin? No? Prove it!

72. There's a reason they called me 'tripod' in college.

73. I give great mammograms. Let's go into my office and I'll show you.

74. I just got dumped, but you made me forget about it.

75. I know I am staring at your breasts, and I know it's rude, but I just can't stop. Forgive me?

76. I'm the easiest person in the room. Are you the second easiest?

77. I could fall madly in bed with you.

78. Just one night, nothing more, and nothing less. You game?

79. You make this room too damn hot - I might have to take off my clothes.

80. I only have cigarettes after sex, and I'm craving one right now.

81. I'm lost in the ocean of those beautiful blue eyes.

82. I'm a genie here to grant three wishes - as long as they involve sex.

83. Pickup lines are lame. Let's just get to the point and fuck.

84. I'll bet you say no to all the guys. But I'm not just another guy.

85. I work as a surgeon. Come back to my place and I'll show you how talented my hands are.

86. All those curves…and I have no brakes.

87. I'm an organ donor. Would you like to play with my organ?

88. Nascar ain't got nothing on those curves of yours.

89. I've got a condom if you've got the time.

90. You make me want to be a better man.

91. My teeth hurt, you're so sweet!

92. You're what I want to see wrapped up underneath my tree this year.

93. Have you ever had anal sex? Tonight's your lucky night!

94. That jacket would look great on my bedroom floor.

95. Good thing there are no pirates around - they would be stealing that gorgeous booty!

96. I'm taking applications for girlfriends…want to sign up?

97. Ho hum hum and a bottle of rum - want to join me?

98. Kiss me, I'm Irish. I'm good luck!

99. I have some Viagra…want to help me see if it really works?

100. I don't want to sleep with you. I want to get to

know you.

101. Hello, gorgeous…my name is ____.

101 Places To Have Sex

1. Hotel bed

2. In the Jacuzzi

3. On top of a fire truck

4. In the pouring rain

5. In front of the mirror

6. On a golf cart

7. On the carpeted staircase

8. On the front porch swing

9. In a classroom after everyone has gone home

10. Backseat of your car

11. Drive-in Movie Theater (in the back row!)

12. Bedroom

13. In a canoe

14. On top of a pool table

15. Laundry room on top of the washer

16. Airplane bathroom

17. Back row of the movie theater

18. At a concert among the crush of fans

19. On the Ferris wheel (you have to be fast!)

20. At the airport terminal

21. In the back aisles of the superstore

22. On your childhood bed during a family reunion

23. In the snow

24. In a furniture store

25. On a tractor

26. In the living room floor

27. In a Porta-Potty at the big concert event (this tests your bravery, too!)

28. On the kitchen table

29. Under the stars in the backyard

30. On a mountaintop in the middle of a hike

31. In your office at work

32. On your boss's desk

33. On a boat in the middle of the ocean

34. In the ocean itself

35. On the beach

36. While in the tanning bed

37. In the lighted pool at night

38. In the center of an ice-skating rink

39. On the riding lawn mower

40. Under the fireworks on the Fourth of July

41. On a hotel balcony

42. In an elevator (again, how fast are you?)

43. Up against a tree in the woods

44. While in an old-fashioned phone booth

45. In the changing room at the department store

46. Among the old forgotten shelves at the library

47. On the golf course (18th hole, of course)

48. In front of your live webcam

49. At the Playboy mansion (hey, why not?)

50. Under a waterfall

51. In an antique shop on an antique bed

52. In a sleeping bag while camping

53. While standing up in the shower

54. While under the blanket at the big football game

55. While going through the car wash

56. On your parents' bed

57. At a basketball game under the stands

58. In a corn maze in autumn

59. At the zoo

60. Under a highway overpass

61. In the middle of the football field in the middle of the night

62. While talking on the phone

63. Underneath the Christmas tree

64. On the hood of your car

65. In a haunted house during Halloween - wear your masks!

66. On the subway

67. In an old barn

68. While in the back of a limousine

69. On the train

70. On a cruise ship, up against the rail

71. In the quietest corner of a museum

72. On a stage during a live sex show

73. In front of your friends

74. On a street corner (don't get caught!)

75. At your desk while working

76. On a picnic table at the park

77. On the big table in the conference room

78. While stuck in a traffic jam

79. On your favorite recliner

80. In a secluded corner of the casino floor

81. While on horseback

82. In a hammock in the backyard

83. On the riverbank

84. Behind the stage during a concert

85. On the band's tour bus

86. On the roof of your house (be careful!)

87. While on a sight-seeing tour on a helicopter

88. While in a hot air balloon

89. In a photography studio (while the camera captures it all)

90. On set for an amateur porn movie

91. In the aisles of the hardware store

92. In the car you are test driving

93. On the side of the road

94. In the bathroom stall

95. In the bed of a pickup truck

96. In the private jet

97. At a highway rest area

98. In a cave

99. At the gym on one of the machines

100. On a motorcycle

101. On a pier just above the crashing waves

DIRTY TALK COLLECTION – BOOK 1

101 Places To Meet Single

1. Your favorite local bar

2. The hotel lounge

3. A wild dance club

4. At the next cubicle over at work

5. At the hobby shop

6. On the treadmill at the gym

7. While volunteering in a third-world country

8. In the co-ed sauna

9. On the Habitat for Humanity crew

10. Through a matchmaker

11. While attending the company picnic

12. Through a friend's introduction

13. Your best friend's party

14. At the doctor's office

15. The company after-hours mixer

16. At antique auctions

17. A community Christmas party

18. The local convenience store

19. While camping in the middle of nowhere

20. During your acting class

21. At the shop where you buy your camping gear

22. The grocery store

23. While on a business trip

24. A Christian youth group

25. On Facebook

26. During happy hour

27. Your favorite Church during Sunday evening service

28. Over the internet

29. During an internet chat

30. Over the telephone

31. At a festival

32. While wandering the fairgrounds

33. On the back roads while riding your ATV

34. In first class on your next flight

35. Cigar clubs

36. Single parent dating clubs

37. On a nature trail

38. During the annual college bonfire

39. In the motorcycle club

40. While attending a charity event at an expensive restaurant

41. At the office where your best friend works

42. On an online dating site

43. While speed dating

44. Through a phone sex hotline

45. When stopping at a charity car wash

46. During a tour of Italy

47. At your local wine tasting event

48. From the personals ads in the back of the paper

49. On Craigslist

50. During language classes

51. While you are taking your boat out for a sail

52. At the animal shelter

53. While dining at a restaurant

54. Picking up your dress from the dry cleaner's shop

55. At your kid's dance recital

56. At the choir performance

57. While attending a summer workshop

58. Doing clothes at The Laundromat

59. While throwing a Frisbee to your cute-as-a-button dog

60. At the ice cream parlor

61. While playing with your kids at the water park

62. While walking along a downtown street

63. At a concert

64. While cheering on your favorite baseball team

65. During your cooking class

66. Mailing packages at the Post Office

67. While playing blackjack at the casino

68. During a movie on the beach

69. At the beach while surfing

70. At the golf course

71. While walking your dog in the park

72. At the high school reunion

73. In your favorite support group

74. While babysitting your friend's kid

75. On the racquetball court

76. During a political rally

77. At the open house at your child's school

78. At a drive-in movie

79. While playing at the arcade

80. In the darkness of a theater

81. During the charity basketball game

82. At the football stadium

83. At the pool

84. The quiet art museum

85. Beside the park fountain on a very hot day

86. While standing at the concession stand

87. At Mardi Gras!

88. At the fast food joint

89. In your college class

90. At your fraternity or sorority party

91. At your best friend's wedding

92. During your graduation party

93. While attending your study group in the library

94. At the bookstore

95. At a book club meeting

96. At a reading or book signing

97. At the coffee house while sipping cappuccino

98. During your vacation in Mexico

99. On a single's cruise to the islands

100. At the neighborhood barbeque

101. When you least expect it!

101 Signs Of A Cheating Partner

1. Your partner is acting strange and distant.

2. They suddenly have new friends they want to spend more time with.

3. You find an email account you never knew they had.

4. They often come home late at night and aren't hungry for dinner.

5. Their old friends seem to have disappeared.

6. They hang up the phone as soon as you walk into the room.

7. They run out to the store for frivolous things that could have waited.

8. They bring home extravagant gifts for no reason.

9. You stumble upon email correspondence that leads you to a dating site.

10. They are always too tired for sex.

11. You see strange numbers on the phone bill.

12. They never answer the phone in their hotel room while they are away.

13. They erase all messages and missed calls from their phone history.

14. They don't flirt with you or respond to your

advances any longer.

15. They get a parking ticket from a place they shouldn't have been.

16. You find cologne or perfume in the glove compartment of their car.

17. Someone who doesn't smoke suddenly smells like cigarettes when they come home.

18. They ask their cell phone provider to stop itemizing their calls.

19. They clear the history on the computer every day.

20. They start talking in terms of "what if" and suggesting that things might change in the future.

21. They find a good reason to storm out of the house to "clear their head."

22. They play on the internet much more often.

23. They want to spend less time as a family and more time alone.

24. Their friends begin avoiding you.

25. They say they work overtime, but their checks don't reflect more pay.

26. There are strange ATM withdrawals on the account.

27. Their body language is evasive.

28. They can't look you in the eye anymore.

29. You find Viagra hidden in his briefcase.

30. When you ask where they have been, their answers sound rehearsed.

31. Someone runs into them while they are with someone else, and calls to tell you.

32. Your phone rings but when you answer, the person hangs up.

33. Odd charges pop up on the credit card bill.

34. They put distance between you when you are both in the same room.

35. They begin using instant messenger when they had no need for it before.

36. They pick fights over little things that make no sense.

37. Your friends begin dropping hints about your partner's faithfulness.

38. They don't answer their cell phone when you call.

39. As soon as they pull out of the driveway, they start making calls on their cell phone.

40. When they call back, they are annoyed that you called in the first place.

41. They come home smelling like a fresh shower.

42. They start wearing sexy lingerie or switch from boxers to briefs.

43. He takes off his wedding band.

44. She suddenly has a new piece of expensive jewelry.

45. You find condoms in the glove compartment.

46. They have a sudden interest in new sexual fetishes.

47. They get upset if you answer their cell phone.

48. They call you by someone else's name.

49. They come home smelling of a body wash you have never bought for them.

50. They stay up late or get up early to use the computer in private.

51. They take business trips more frequently than ever.

52. They lose interest in having sex with you.

53. Vacations and longer trips always seem to get canceled at the last minute.

54. She is suddenly very concerned with birth control methods.

55. They encourage you to take a trip alone.

56. They seem to mention one particular person work more than others.

57. You smell perfume or cologne that is not you

when you walk into your house, as though someone has been
there…but your partner denies it.

58. You are no longer invited along on business trips.

59. You find condom wrappers under the bed -- but you don't use condoms.

60. They get defensive when you ask them a question.

61. They shut down internet windows very quickly when you walk into a room.

62. The radio in the car is set to a station neither of you ever listen to.

63. They have suddenly used up all their vacation days, but they didn't use them with you.

64. Your partner suddenly breaks out the new moves in bed.

65. You find love notes in their pocket.

66. The children mention your partner's "special friend."

67. You find a receipt for a hotel or restaurant you have never visited.

68. Your partner shows up with love bites or scratches on their body.

69. They seem to be looking for something you might do wrong.

70. They ridicule you for questioning whether they are faithful.

71. Their boss calls looking for them -- but they told YOU they were on a business trip for the company.

72. They are suddenly confident about everything and walk with a bounce in their step.

73. They seem very suspicious of you for no reason at all.

74. The thought of taking a vacation makes them depressed rather than happy.

75. Your partner purchases prepaid phone cards when they have a working cell phone.

76. He suddenly wants to do all the laundry.

77. She has new lingerie that she never wears for you.

78. The mileage on the car says they didn't drive to the office -- they drove out of town.

79. They aren't registered at the hotel they told you they would be staying at for the conference.

80. You find unusual stains on their clothes.

81. They suddenly ask you for an open relationship.

82. A certain someone leaves flirty messages on the Facebook or MySpace page.

83. Your partner makes your bed with fresh sheets every few days -- but they never bothered to make the be

before.

84. Their car smells like someone else's perfume or cologne.

85. The GPS in the car shows an unusual address.

86. They claim to play golf every Saturday, but their golf bags haven't been moved.

87. You find flirty text messages on their phone.

88. The passenger seat is often in a strange position - certainly not the one you left it in!

89. They have a post office box for no apparent reason.

90. They want to know where you are at all times.

91. She suddenly wants a makeover and new clothes.

92. You come home early and catch them with their lover.

93. He starts going to the tanning bed.

94. You catch them in a lie, and they tell another lie to get out of it.

95. You get an interesting email from someone who claims to be your partner's new lover.

96. A gym membership becomes the most important thing in the world.

97. You go to the doctor and discover you have an STD…but you have been with ONLY your partner.

98. They panic when you tell them and try to blame you.

99. You discover a secret savings account.

100. You mention your concerns and your partner accuses you of being crazy.

101. Your gut tells you something is wrong -- and you can't shake that feeling.

101 Things To Never Do In Bed

1. Say someone else's name

2. Slap your lover around (unless they want it!)

3. Talk about your exes

4. Criticize

5. Ask "Is that it?"

6. Laugh at the size of his penis

7. Tell her you can't feel the walls of her vagina when you fuck

8. Invite his best friend without his permission

9. Tell her your momma fantasy

10. Ask her if she wants to do the dog

11. Call out the name of your brother when you cum

12. Shoot your cum into her eye

13. Shoot it into her hair

14. Rip your partner's thousand-dollar teddy

15. Start crying about your car payment

16. Think about baseball stats

17. Slide it into the wrong hole

18. Get it on with her mom

19. Have at it with his dad

20. Suck off the wrong person while blindfolded

21. Invite a complete stranger for unsafe sex

22. Puncture the condom

23. Lie about your herpes condition

24. Stop taking your birth control without telling him

25. Ignore your lover

26. Tell them they are a filthy slut – and mean it

27. Kiss like a monkey slobbering

28. Go straight for the naughty bits with no foreplay

29. Acting like a child who wants to suck mommy's tits

30. Deep throating with a serious gag reflex

31. Bite hard enough to draw blood

32. Asking why she doesn't like your moves, because her sister sure did!

33. Shove all your fingers into her with no warm-up

34. Stopping when he begs you to keep going

35. Allowing no safe word

36. Expect your partner to shave just because you like it

37. Come to bed unclean

38. Suffocate your partner to the point of passing out

39. Fart in their face

40. Go down on her, only to complain about the taste

41. Insist he go down on you during your period

42. Forget and leave the tampon in

43. Blame her if you can't get it up

44. Drink too much and then forget where the hole is

45. Hold her head down while you cum – and she can't breathe

46. Talk about her mother's tits while you're fucking her

47. Call her your daughter if she's not into role-play

48. Tell him how cute his little dicky-wicky is

49. Get out the measuring tape

50. Tell jokes about vaginas the size of 747s

51. Ask "How many kids did you say you had?"

52. Make her gag on your cock just because you like the

power trip

53. Talk about the size of his penis... unless it's a good size!

54. Cum too fast and then go to sleep

55. Even worse, fall asleep during sex

56. Fuck when you're both feeling a bit under the weather

57. Come in her mouth without asking first

58. Bite down on him while giving a blowjob

59. Expect your partner to fuck like a porn star

60. Tell him you bet his best buddy is hung like a horse

61. Ask her to fuck her best friend while you watch

62. Turn on a hardcore porn film without discussing it first

63. Answer the phone during sex

64. Videotape anything without permission

65. Break out the hardcore heavy shit, like you grandpa's knife

66. Make him do all the work while you lay there like fish

67. Compare him to your ex

68. Go up her backdoor by "accident"

69. Keep up the same old boring routine

70. Get mad at her when she talks dirty to you

71. Shove sweet fruits into her vagina and then forget to lick them out

72. Let the dog or cat watch you going at it

73. Spank her out of the blue

74. Break out the strap on without discussing the idea

75. Forget the romance

76. Avoid the cuddle time

77. Forget to clean up after you're done

78. Ask him to lick his own cum out of you

79. Cum on her without asking her first

80. Shoot your cum into her without making sure it's okay

81. Invite a friend back to your place when he wants to play

82. Have an affair

83. Tell him he reminds you of your father

84. Have sex with your partner while another man's cum is still inside you – unless you're kinky like that

84. Squeeze his balls to make him slow down

86. Always use your vibrator

87. Get him hot and bothered and then say "not tonight"

88. Collapse on her without regard for whether she can breathe

89. Yell at him but don't tell him what he did wrong

90. Call her a bitch or a cunt before she tells you it's okay to do so

91. Scream right in his ear when you cum

92. Tell him you are fantasizing that he is someone else

93. Forget how to find the g-spot

94. Poke around like a virgin during his first time

95. Be bashful about opening up your sexual horizons

96. Stroke your partner in a way that causes pain, not pleasure

97. Stick foreign objects into sexual orifices – unless you're both kinky like that

98. Take that phone call in the middle of intercourse

99. Pay attention to the game on television instead of her

100. Tell her she needs to lose weight

101. Ask him "Is it in yet?"

101 Ultra Kinky Sex Ideas

1. Tie your partner up and break out the vibrator.

2. Cover each other with oil before slipping and sliding on silk sheets.

3. Get it on in the backyard pool in the middle of the day.

4. Watch kinky porn and imitate the actors.

5. Surprise your partner with a set of anal beads.

6. Go to a sex shop together and choose a new vibrator.

7. Let your best friend watch you fuck your partner.

8. Have a sexual encounter with a member of the same sex.

9. Let your best friend fuck your partner and YOU watch.

10. Pick up a stranger and make out with them.

11. Introduce your man to anal sex - both giving AND receiving.

12. Meet the UPS guy at the door wearing nothing all.

13. Lick chocolate sauce from your lover's body.

14. Call a phone sex hotline and get your sexy on.

15. Dress up as his ultimate fantasy and stay in character all night.

16. Visit a sex club and watch everyone else have sex.

17. Touch your partner from head to toe…only with your breath.

18. Spank your partner while you're fucking them.

19. Get it on while flying on an airplane.

20. Do it on a hotel balcony.

21. Demand all oral sex - and nothing else.

22. Videotape your action.

23. Try out Japanese rope bondage.

24. Come all over your lover's face.

25. Pull your lover's hair as they are coming.

26. Wait on the bed for your lover wearing nothing at all.

27. Bend over a chair and invite your partner to take you.

28. Invite a photographer into the room to capture your lovemaking.

29. Wear high heels to bed.

30. Make your lover dress up in your clothes.

31. Explore domination and submission.

32. Blindfold your partner and make them guess who is fucking them. You - or someone else?

33. Suck on your lover's balls while he jacks off.

34. Masturbate in front of your partner.

35. Slide your cock between her breasts and fuck her that way.

36. Take photographs of each other to post on the internet.

37. Butt plugs are an ass lover's best friend.

38. Lead your lover around by a leash.

39. Stay naked at home all day and have sex as often as possible.

40. Lube yourself up, spread your cheeks, and invite your partner to take your ass.

41. Go through every position in the Kama Sutra.

42. Invest in nipple clamps and let the games begin!

43. Clothespins provide pressure on delicate body parts - try it!

44. Give your partner head while they are driving.

45. Suck on your lover's toes while they are tied up.

46. Try out a double-ended dildo.

47. Get right on the edge of orgasm…but don't let each other come all night long.

48. Wear bright red lipstick as your suck your partner's cock.

49. Surprise your partner with quickie sex at work.

50. Convince your partner to wear your lingerie.

51. Keep your panties on while you fuck.

52. Wear leather outfits while you go at it.

53. Get a riding crop from the sex toy store and "ride" your partner with it.

54. Get a vibrator with a remote and go out on the town together.

55. Do it in your old childhood bedroom.

56. Fuck your lover in the public Jacuzzi at a hotel.

57. "Torture" your lover with ice all over their body.

58. Ask your lover to suck another man's cock.

59. Do the nasty in the snow!

60. Have sex in the same room with another couple and watch each other.

61. Purchase the largest dildo you can find and see how much of it she can take.

62. Take a class on striptease and then surprise your partner.

63. Find his prostate and massage it until he comes.

64. Use sex toys to fill up every hole.

65. Slide pieces of fruit into your lover's pussy and suck them out.

66. Before you have anal sex, give your partner an enema.

67. Slip your finger up your man's ass right as he's about to come.

68. Threaten to fuck him hard up the ass if he doesn't make you come properly!

69. Drip soy-wax cool candles all over your partner's body.

70. Use Pop Rocks to give your lover a sexy, bubbly sensation as you go down.

71. Hire a man or woman from an escort service and play to your heart's content.

72. Compete to see who can come first.

73. Fuck each other in a mirrored room.

74. Have "sliding sex" by lying down a shower curtain on the floor and covering each other with olive oil.

75. Explore needle play - especially on the nipples.

76. Spank your partner with a hairbrush.

77. Watch two men go at it - or two women, whatever floats your boat.

78. Have sex in the parking lot of the sex toy store.

79. Pick up a stranger and have sex with them while your lover watches.

80. Make your partner wear a cock ring that will make him last longer.

81. Make a point of fucking for as long as you can - the point is to be sore as hell in the morning!

82. Go down on a man in a crowded place, like a bar.

83. After you've come inside your woman, lick your own come out of her.

84. Pretend to be a cop picking up a prostitute, and do it in a public park.

85. If he comes in your mouth, kiss him when he's done.

86. Use toys to find her g-spot and see what you can do with it!

87. Do your Kegel exercises while he is inside you.

88. Get your tongue pierced to give your lover a more sensual thrill.

89. Use a penis extender to give your woman a little

something more.

90. Become your partner's sex slave for an evening.

91. Dress up in some of the kinkier fetishes - horse and rider is a good one.

92. Host an "interrogation" - tie your partner up and "torture" them with pleasures as they answer naughty questions.

93. Use a toy that offers a tiny electrical jolt on your partner.

94. Get a sensual tattoo on one of your most delicate body parts.

95. Get a "pocket pussy" for him and fulfill that fantasy of having more than one pussy at a time…

96. Give someone their first gay or lesbian experience.

97. Invest in sex furniture, like the Liberator.

98. Explore her body and try to make her "squirt" when she comes.

99. With more than one man? Let them all come on your body and cover you with it.

100. Have sex standing up in the shower.

101. Ask your partner what their deepest, darkest fantasy is…and make it happen!

101 Ways To Capture His Heart

1. Cook him something that he will never forget.

2. Give the best blowjobs ever.

3. Send flowers to him at work.

4. Tell your friends how much you love him.

5. Call him for no reason at all.

6. Send him a card with hearts.

7. Buy him a dog.

8. Wear something naughty for him.

9. Save his picture to your screensaver.

10. Take him on a romantic trip.

11. Let him work on your car.

12. Become friends with his mother.

13. Mix a CD of love songs just for him.

14. Come to bed dressed in his favorite team's jersey.

15. Learn all about his favorite sport.

16. Get tickets to his favorite sporting event.

17. Let him sit on the couch with a beer and his buddies all day.

18. Learn how to bait your own hook and take him fishing.

19. Cook a steak for him – and another for his dog.

20. Wash his truck in your bikini.

21. Put in a porn film without him having to ask.

22. Get him a subscription to Hustler.

23. Send him to the sex toy shop with instructions to buy something naughty for you.

24. Slip a love note into his briefcase.

25. Send him a sultry email detailing your fantasies.

26. Never talk about your exes in his presence.

27. Put a post-it note on his mirror telling him about what body part you like best.

28. Teach him what the male g-spot is.

29. Leave a voicemail telling him you are thinking about him.

30. Record yourself having an orgasm and give him the CD.

31. Set up the video camera and make it even more vivid!

32. Meet him at the door wrapped in only his shirt.

33. Tie him to the bed and take over for an evening.

34. Make a cast dildo of his cock to use while he is away.

35. Surprise him on that business trip by showing up in his room in a negligee.

36. Call him for phone sex while he's at work.

37. Come up with new and inventive ways to make phone sex feel more like the real thing.

38. Tuck a pair of your panties into his glove compartment for him to find later.

39. Make him your "last call" of the day, every day.

40. Dress up like a stripper and pretend you're someone else for a night.

41. Take a stripping class and learn how to polish his pole in more ways than one.

42. Learn how to belly dance.

43. Take him to the store with you to pick out your spring and summer wardrobe.

44. Let him choose his favorite swimsuit or bikini for you.

45. Trail roses all over his body.

46. Let him have anal sex with you.

47. Better yet, teach him how good it can be to receive

anal sex!

48. Cook a romantic dinner for him.

49. Fuck him outside underneath the stars.

50. Play footsie with his dick under the restaurant tablecloth.

51. Suck on that ice cream cone tell him it will soon be him.

52. Mow his lawn while he's at work.

53. Invite your best friend for a threesome and make him the focus of the action.

54. Ask him to star in his very own porn film.

55. Serve him luscious fruits with your body as the plate.

56. Wear edible underwear for a nice surprise.

57. Buy a book of naughty positions and try them one by one.

58. Write an erotic story for him.

59. Read that story to him while you are in bed together.

60. Learn the thrill of getting mud on the tires!

61. Plan a campout in the bed of his truck.

62. Put a picture of him on your desk at work.

63. Surprise him with an impromptu flight to his favorite city.

64. Join the mile-high club!

65. Listen to what he has to say.

66. Remember the names of his friends and the kind of beer they like.

67. Give him a pet name.

68. Don't pressure him into anything at all – let him be the one that makes that call.

69. Invite him to a game of strip poker.

70. Take him to strip club for his birthday and buy him a lap dance.

71. Better yet, buy yourself a lap dance and let him watch.

72. Raid his kitchen for sex toys – dinner will never be the same.

73. Kiss him on the Ferris Wheel and make him feel like a kid again.

74. Go necking in the back of his prized classic car.

75. Give him a hickey to show off to his friends.

76. Give him a written list of all the things you love about him.

77. Take your farmer boy to the barn and do it in hayloft.

78. Give him public displays of affection.

79. Take him to church and whisper naughty thoughts into his ear throughout the sermon.

80. Learn about all the things he is interested in.

81. Leave fresh-baked cookies in his kitchen.

82. Always have your fridge stocked with his favorite

83. Give him a key to your place.

84. Ask him to make love to you on his prized boat.

85. Meet him in a hotel for a lunchtime quickie.

86. Take him to see an action movie instead of a chick flick.

87. Invest in a dozen thongs and ask him to choose which ones you wear on any given day.

88. Get in the shower with him to soap him up.

89. Draw a sweet bubble bath and ride him like a whore while you're in it.

90. Pretend you're a virgin and ask him to teach you the ways of the world.

91. Make a point of getting to know his father.

92. Write a poem about him.

93. Write about your love for him on your blog.

94. Change your Facebook status to "in a relationship."

95. Tell him he's the only one you will ever want.

96. Give him a long, thorough massage from head to toe.

97. Ask him if you're in his future.

98. Burn your little black book.

99. Turn convention on its head and propose to him.

100. Call a radio station and dedicate a love song to him.

101. Tell him you want to bear his children.

101 Ways To Come Out Of The Closet

1. Write a coming out letter.

2. Change your status on Facebook.

3. Refuse to label yourself or anyone else.

4. Go on a date with a member of the same sex and let your friends see you together.

5. Send a video to your family explaining your sexuality.

6. Tell your most trusted friend, then ask them to help you tell others.

7. Start a blog to announce it to the world.

8. Hit up MySpace and surprise your friends with the announcement.

9. Tell your family and friends in private.

10. Think long and hard about who to tell first.

11. Get a divorce from your straight spouse and hook up with your gay friend.

12. Give your friends and family books on gay marriage.

13. Never apologize for who you are!

14. Have an "escape plan" for the aftermath.

15. Say it in a firm, loud voice.

16. Have sex with someone who gossips and will spread the news all over town.

17. Tell them you will still be gay no matter what their response might be.

18. Take the time to answer all their questions.

19. Let your best friend do the talking while you make yourself scarce.

20. Write it in graffiti on your wall.

21. Go on a gay cruise.

22. Tell someone over a nice dinner.

23. Let someone find your same-sex porn collection.

24. Wait until your birthday and start the new year of your life the right way.

25. Go to a gay club and invite your friends.

26. Mention how much you like the same sex when you're in bed with your spouse.

27. Tell the world on Twitter.

28. Let your attorney tell them when you serve the divorce papers.

29. Be prepared to leave the person alone for a while after you come out to them.

30. Come out to only one person at a time.

31. Move into that one-bedroom apartment with your "best friend."

32. Send a long email explaining your sexuality.

33. Role-play "gay" games until your spouse gets the picture.

34. Bring home your new partner for the holidays.

35. Let your partner find the sex toys you have kept hidden.

36. Ask your family how they feel about homosexuality, and take it from there.

37. Yell it from the rooftops.

38. Come out only if everyone is sober.

39. Let incriminating photos of you leak onto the web.

40. Be prepared to hear absolutely anything in response to the news.

41. Never come out while arguing with someone.

42. Let the rumors start, and don't bother to correct them.

43. Propose to your gay lover in public.

44. Never come out while under the influence of drugs or alcohol.

45. Bring your partner to the family reunion.

46. Wait until someone asks, and then come out to them.

47. Come out in drag!

48. Join the march for gay rights.

49. Wear flamboyant clothing that leaves no doubt of your orientation.

50. Start a discussion about orientation at the dinner table.

51. Say it in a text message.

52. Don't come out in a moving car.

53. Keep a "coming out" journal and let your friends read it when it's full.

54. Invite your family and friends to your wedding.

55. Argue loudly for gay marriage rights and then explain why.

56. Compare yourself to an openly gay celebrity.

57. Recognize that coming out is a process, not a one-time event.

58. Fly the rainbow flag from your front porch.

59. Tell everyone on National Coming Out Day.

60. Leave pamphlets about coming out on your living

room table for visitors to see.

61. Come out on television.

62. Come out during a gay pride parade.

63. Put a rainbow sticker on the back of your car.

64. Come out by taking your friends to a gay movie theater.

65. Rent "Brokeback Mountain" to get the discussion started.

66. Explain that you're still the same person -- you just have a different orientation.

67. Come out on a talk show.

68. Write a book about your sexuality.

69. Don't fight who you are!

70. Don't be surprised if your family and friends knew already.

71. Get comfortable with your sexuality before you discuss it with anyone.

72. Don't get offended by questions.

73. Leave a site on coming out open on your computer when you have company.

74. Give your phone number to that person you've always been attracted to.

75. Offer phone numbers to gay and lesbian hotlines for those who have trouble with your announcement.

76. Be prepared to feel overwhelmed by the questions.

77. Stay away from hateful people.

78. Don't push anyone to accept your coming out, but express how much you hope they will come around.

79. Write down what you want to say before you have "the talk."

80. Reassure your friends and family that you are taking good care of your health.

81. Be prepared to dispel any myths that might be brought up.

82. Know that it might take time before some people believe you.

83. Round up a good support group before you start to come out of the closet.

84. Don't worry about finding the right time. When it's time, you will know.

85. Say what you need to say in a phone call.

86. Put a video on You Tube and send the link to everyone who needs to see it.

87. Wear a "gay pride" bracelet.

88. Understand all the terms associated with the LGBT community.

89. Explain that you don't have all the answers -- you're still figuring it out.

90. Ask for your friends and family to help you through the coming out process.

91. Recognize that love comes in many forms.

92. Wait for someone to ask about your orientation.

93. Say it on the front of a t-shirt.

94. Browse the gay erotica section of the bookstore.

95. Leave gay erotica novels on the bedside table.

96. Plan to sit down and discuss your orientation for hours

97. Understand that coming out might put some distance between you and your loved ones for a while.

98. Come out over the public intercom at the airport.

99. Come out at your high school reunion.

100. Come out only to those whose opinion matters t you.

101. Remember that coming out takes trust -- ar remind your loved ones of how much that trust means you.

101 Ways To Flirt

1. Talk in a low, quiet tone.

2. Deepen your voice if you can.

3. When there is a pause in the conversation, fill it with a smile.

4. Hold eye contact.

5. Give him or her your full attention.

6. Look at her out of the corner of your eye, then look away.

7. Leave the drama at home.

8. If you want to break the ice, learn a neat magic trick.

9. Ask an off-beat question that gets attention fast.

10. Follow the cues you get back. If they are interested, you will know.

11. Wear clothes that show off your best assets.

12. Walk very slowly toward the object of your affection.

13. Play with her hair.

14. Tease him by playing with his collar.

15. Twirl your fingertip around a button on their shirt.

16. Accuse him or her of flirting with you. It always

brings a smile!

17. Blow a kiss from across the room.

18. Send a drink with your compliments.

19. Write your phone number on a napkin and tuck it into his pocket.

20. Play with your straw or seductively sip the ice from your glass.

21. Use sexual innuendo to get attention.

22. Pay attention to what they say to you - that gets you noticed!

23. Let her use you. Does she have trouble reaching the item on the top shelf of the grocery store? Swoop in and get it for you, then introduce yourself.

24. Tailor your comments to the situation at hand.

25. Don't be afraid to invade personal space.

26. Ask mundane questions followed by fun comments. For example, if you ask where she's from and she tells you she's from Alabama, remind her of how sexy southern accents are!

27. Accuse her of being naughty.

28. Tell her she's beautiful - and mean it.

29. If you are really into him, ask him if you could go someplace quieter.

30. Touch his hand to show him you're interested in contact.

31. Have interesting comments ready - people absolutely love useless trivia.

32. Read up on human sexuality and be prepared with interesting facts.

33. Use double-meanings every time you can manage to get them into the conversation.

34. Give her a nickname right off the bat.

35. Lift your eyebrow when you make a fun point.

36. Stand between her and the crowd so she notices only you.

37. When you go for a walk, move slowly.

38. If it's chilly, put your jacket around her shoulders.

39. Walking along the beach or on grass? Offer to carry her high heels for her.

40. Casually lick your lips as you look at him.

41. When you sit down, cross your legs toward him - that's a big sign that you're interested.

42. Laugh at her jokes and tell a few of your own.

43. Look right at her, even if you're talking to someone else.

44. Lift your glass in appreciation when she looks your

way.

45. Follow her around the room and when she looks at you, tell her that you thought she was following you!

46. Walk right up to her friend and ask them to introduce you.

47. Speak softly so he has to lean in to hear you.

48. Never, ever speak of exes, your mother, or anything else that might lead to negative thoughts on her part. Focus on her and only her.

49. Make yourself interesting! Read the newspaper and stay up-to-date on current events.

50. Avoid talking about religion or politics unless she brings it up first.

51. Give her sincere compliments.

52. Tell her you like the way you can make her blush.

53. If you're comfortable talking to him, tell him so.

54. Be confident. If you walk in with a sexy swagger and mean it, she will be more attracted to you.

55. Lower your chin and look up at him. This pose makes him feel more powerful and attractive.

56. Ask him if he's coming onto you. If he says yes, respond with "Good." If he says no, respond with "Well, what are you waiting for?"

57. Be a bit sarcastic…many people like that wry sense

of humor.

58. Allude to sex with every other comment. If he says he likes to play football, ask him something like, "So you like the rough games, do you?"

59. Send him a drink with a suggestive name, like a Fuzzy Navel or a Sex on the Beach.

60. Flat-out ask what they love about sex. That makes it clear where your mind is headed!

61. Slide your hand down her shoulder.

62. Touch her hand, hold it for a moment, then let it go.

63. Use shameless props. If someone comes up to you while you are walking your dog in the park, tell her you hoped he would be a chick magnet...then hold out your hand and introduce yourself.

64. Be spontaneous and go with the flow.

65. Straighten his tie - or better yet, loosen it.

66. If you're the shy type, admit it! Women love honesty from the very beginning.

67. Ask her, "Please tell me you're alone tonight...it will break my heart if you're with someone!"

68. If you do get the brush off, be courteous, smile, and back off. She will remember that you were a gentleman - and so will her friends, who might very well be available!

69. Be selective - flirt with someone only if you mean it.

If they have seen you flirting with half the room before you get to them, they won't be interested, no matter how smooth you are.

70. When you say goodbye, kiss her hand before you go.

71. No paper about? Write your number on her hand.

72. Place your hand on the small of her back as you walk through a crowd. It makes women swoon.

73. Brush "lint" from his jacket to get closer to him.

74. Pickup lines are for amateurs.

75. Can you get her to dance? Good! That gives you the opportunity to get even closer.

76. If she is sitting down, stand with one foot slightly between hers.

77. If he's sitting down, ease onto his lap with a mischievous smile.

78. Remember who you flirt with. The last thing you want is a call from a woman who is really interested, but you can't remember where you met or what you talked about!

79. Acknowledge what you're doing. Saying "I just love to flirt, don't you?" takes away the coy games.

80. Lean over and tap your cheek for a tiny kiss.

81. Slide your hand along her knee.

82. Ask her, "Am I flirting too much?"

83. Undo the top button on your shirt.

84. Share interesting stories about your life experiences.

85. Whisper into her ear.

86. Don't give away everything at once - leave him wanting more!

87. Ask for her number, and call it five minutes later, with the line, "I've waited as long as I could. Want to meet me outside so we can go for a cup of coffee?"

88. If you're at a club, request that the DJ play a song for her. "Pretty Woman" is always good!

89. Look over your shoulder as you walk away from him.

90. Watch her the whole time she's walking away.

91. Practice makes perfect! The more you flirt, the easier it will be.

92. Don't play hard to get. Despite what the dating books say, it doesn't work if you're looking for someone to really connect with. If you're just looking for sex, however, have at it.

93. If she kicks off her shoes, immediately massage her feet.

94. Massage his neck and back - it really does work for matters of seduction!

95. Be prepared to accept a "no" just as readily as you would accept a "yes".

96. Stare at her as she puts lipstick on.

97. When you do get her alone, immediately reach for her hand.

98. Tease her friends and talk to them, but keep your eyes on her.

99. Don't carry cards with your number - that's too obvious. But do have a piece of paper or something in your pocket to write hers down.

100. When you do call her up, tease her with something like, "Did you miss me?"

101. Above all, treat your potential date with respect. That's the best calling card you could possibly offer!

101 Ways To Masturbate

1. Alone.

2. With a partner.

3. On the bed.

4. On the kitchen table.

5. While watching porn.

6. During phone sex.

7. While texting with someone.

8. With a vibrator.

9. With your hands down your pants.

10. With your lover's golf clubs. Swing!

11. Naked in your living room.

12. While humping a stuffed animal.

13. In a public restroom.

14. With the wine bottle.

15. With the shower head.

16. While in the bathtub with the fuzzy sponge.

17. With lots of lube.

18. In a room full of people during National Orgasm Day.

19. With your electric toothbrush.

20. In front of your ex-boyfriend.

21. While bopping to the beat of your favorite album.

22. At a concert with a noise-activated vibrator.

23. With the gearshift of your man's car.

24. While she's going down on you.

25. While you are going down on her.

26. With that cool light-saber toy.

27. While riding the jets in the hot tub.

28. While using Altoids for that brisk, tingly feeling.

29. With a set of drumsticks.

30. With a peppermint stick.

31. With pens, pencils, or highlighters.

32. With his remote control.

33. As a goodbye gift to your soon-to-be ex.

34. While on webcam.

35. With a phone set to vibrate.

36. By using the shampoo bottle.

37. While on video.

38. In the sex toy store while trying out the merchandise.

39. While letting someone take pictures of you.

40. With a pocket pussy.

41. In a hotel room with a perfect stranger.

42. With cucumbers, carrots, and any other veggies that look…tasty.

43. With a banana.

44. While watching yourself in the mirror.

45. While pulling on your pierced nipples.

46. With cool-melt soy candle wax.

47. With the candle itself.

48. By aiming water with a turkey baster.

49. By using his come as lube.

50. With a thin water bottle -- chilled, if you like it like that.

51. While riding the arm of a chair.

52. With a large dildo.

53. With a butt plug up your ass.

54. While someone is fucking your ass.

55. By following directions from your Master.

56. As fast and furious as you can.

57. While getting a tattoo.

58. While making your own amateur porn.

59. While in the backyard pool during a pool party.

60. In your childhood bed.

61. Better yet, in your parents' bed.

62. With a popsicle. Chilly!

63. With a warm sock.

64. With nothing but your fingers.

65. By sticking your dick in a melon.

66. With a lot of prostate stimulation.

67. While using lotion.

68. In the middle of a scene with your submissive.

69. During an intense fantasy about your best friend.

70. By sticking your dick between pillows.

71. While your hands are numb with cold.

72. With snow all over your nether regions.

73. While using an anal sex toy.

74. With a sexy blow-up doll.

75. While using urethral sound tubes.

76. By using the "stop and go" method.

77. While twisting your hands gently up and down your shaft.

78. While rubbing your clit with a bit of lube.

79. With a toy placed right against your g-spot.

80. By fucking a fresh apple pie. (Come on, you've seen the movie!)

81. While on a roof above a busy street.

82. On your boyfriend's voice mail.

83. On your boss's desk when he's out of town.

84. While using a penis pump.

85. Finding someone to do it for you.

86. Using a vacuum hose set on low.

87. While spanking your pussy for being a naughty girl!

88. With your girlfriend's panties wrapped around your dick.

89. While wearing a cock ring.

90. While looking at "girlie" magazines.

91. By jacking to the beat of the radio.

92. While taunting your ex about what they can't have anymore.

93. With a bar of soap in the shower.

94. By using the heel of your fuck-me boots.

95. In the passenger seat while your lover is driving.

96. At the restaurant under the table.

97. In the woods, where only the birds can see you.

98. At the movie theater as you lust after the leading man.

99. With a big wad of cash.

100. While getting encouragement from a message board.

101. In front of your biggest crush of all time.

How To Get More Dirty Talk

Did you like what you have read so far?

Are you curious and want more help with spicing up your relationship?

Just sign up for Denise's newsletter over at Dirty Talk 101. Dirty Talk 101 is Denise's online magazine dedicated to talking dirty, relationships, sexting and much more.

VISIT TODAY
http://www.DirtyTalk101.com

ABOUT THE AUTHOR

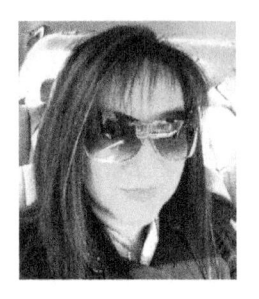

Denise knows relationships very well. She's felt both soaring love and a broken heart. She has had smooth, easy relationships that seemed to be effortless, and she had been in situations where she really had to work hard to sustain the union.

In the depth of those experiences, she has found wha[t] works to sustain and spice up a relationship – and just a[s] importantly, what can lead to a relationship's slow withering demise. Denise combines her real-li[fe] experiences with her passion for writing, and that results [in] novels that are both helpful and hot!

Denise has dozens of novels and ebooks under h[er] saucy leather belt, as well as hundreds of blog posts th[at] showcase her ability to provide the best advice. She is bes[t] known for the wide-ranging "101 Series," in which s[he] pursues everything from getting kinky to romantic g[ift] ideas to what to never, ever do in bed.

But sometimes you just want to read something hot[. If] you are in the mood to ditch the advice and just get y[our] sexy on, check out Denise's erotic short story collection[s]

DIRTY TALK COLLECTION – BOOK 1

Published by

Arrabella Publishing

PO Box 270391

Fort Collins, Colorado 80527

Copyright © 2014 Denise Brienne

All rights reserved.

ISBN: 1499793804
ISBN-13: 978-1499793804

Printed in Great Britain
by Amazon